It's easy to get lost in the cancer world

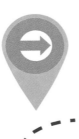

Let **NCCN Guidelines for Patients®** be your guide

✓ Step-by-step guides to the cancer care options likely to have the best results

✓ Based on treatment guidelines used by health care providers worldwide

✓ Designed to help you discuss cancer treatment with your doctors

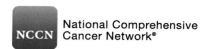

NCCN Guidelines for Patients® are developed by the National Comprehensive Cancer Network® (NCCN®)

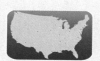

NCCN

✓ An alliance of leading cancer centers across the United States devoted to patient care, research, and education

Cancer centers that are part of NCCN:
NCCN.org/cancercenters

NCCN Clinical Practice Guidelines in Oncology (NCCN Guidelines®)

✓ Developed by doctors from NCCN cancer centers using the latest research and years of experience

✓ For providers of cancer care all over the world

✓ Expert recommendations for cancer screening, diagnosis, and treatment

Free online at
NCCN.org/guidelines

NCCN Guidelines for Patients

✓ Present information from the NCCN Guidelines in an easy-to-learn format

✓ For people with cancer and those who support them

✓ Explain the cancer care options likely to have the best results

Free online at
NCCN.org/patientguidelines

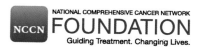

and supported by funding from NCCN Foundation®

These NCCN Guidelines for Patients are based on the NCCN Guidelines® for Pediatric Acute Lymphoblastic Leukemia (Version 1.2021, September 16, 2020).

NCCN Foundation seeks to support the millions of patients and their families affected by a cancer diagnosis by funding and distributing NCCN Guidelines for Patients. NCCN Foundation is also committed to advancing cancer treatment by funding the nation's promising doctors at the center of innovation in cancer research. For more details and the full library of patient and caregiver resources, visit NCCN.org/patients.

National Comprehensive Cancer Network (NCCN) / NCCN Foundation
3025 Chemical Road, Suite 100
Plymouth Meeting, PA 19462
215.690.0300

Endorsed by

Alex's Lemonade Stand Foundation

We at Alex's Lemonade Stand Foundation are honored to endorse the NCCN Guidelines for Patients: Pediatric ALL. We know firsthand how important it is for families to have accurate and trusted information about their child's treatment plan. There is so much power and hope in information!

alexslemonade.org

Be The Match®

National Marrow Donor Program® (NMDP)/Be The Match® is the global leader in providing a possible cure to patients with life-threatening blood and marrow cancers, as well as other diseases. Our Be The Match Patient Support Center provides support, information, and resources for patients, caregivers, and families.

BeTheMatch.org/one-on-one

CancerFree Kids

CancerFree KIDS does ONE thing: we invest in innovative research on childhood cancers to give every kid a chance to grow up. We proudly support the NCCN Foundation's mission to improve the care of children with cancer with these guidelines.

cancerfreekids.org

Pediatric Cancer Foundation of the Lehigh Valley

Pediatric Cancer Foundation of the Lehigh Valley is thrilled to be able to share this valuable resource with our local pediatric cancer families as they navigate their journey with both us and NCCN by their side!

pcflv.org

The Leukemia & Lymphoma Society

The Leukemia & Lymphoma Society (LLS) is dedicated to developing better outcomes for blood cancer patients and their families through research, education, support and advocacy and is happy to have this comprehensive resource available to patients.

lls.org/informationspecialists

To make a gift or learn more, please visit NCCNFoundation.org/donate or e-mail PatientGuidelines@nccn.org.

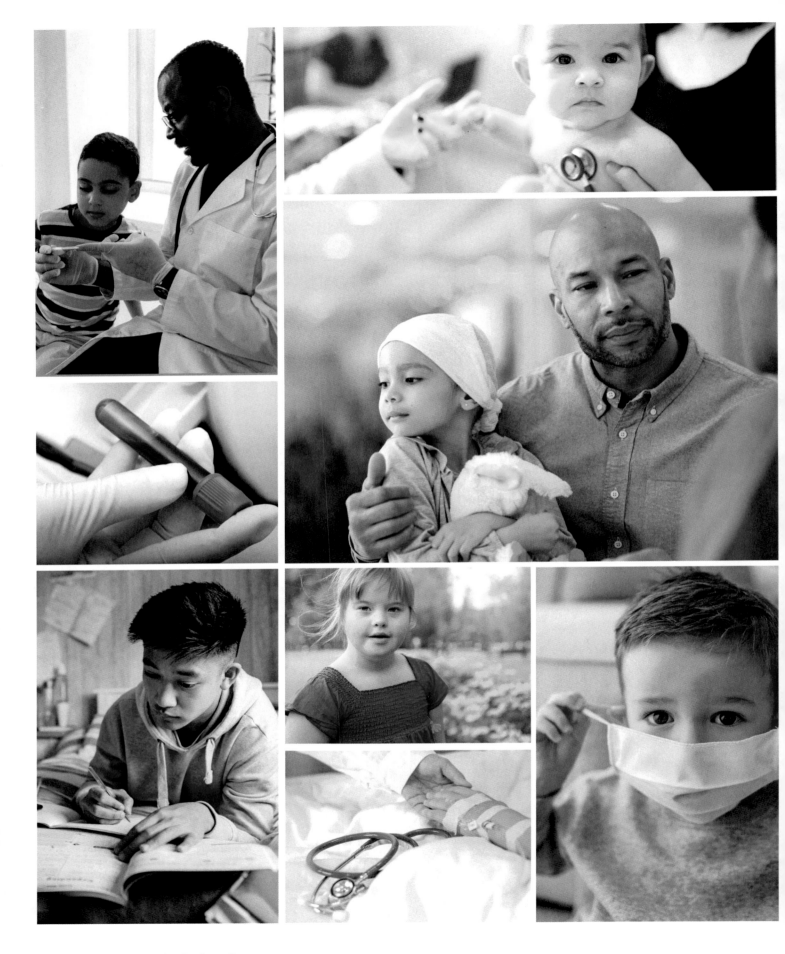

Contents

1
ALL basics

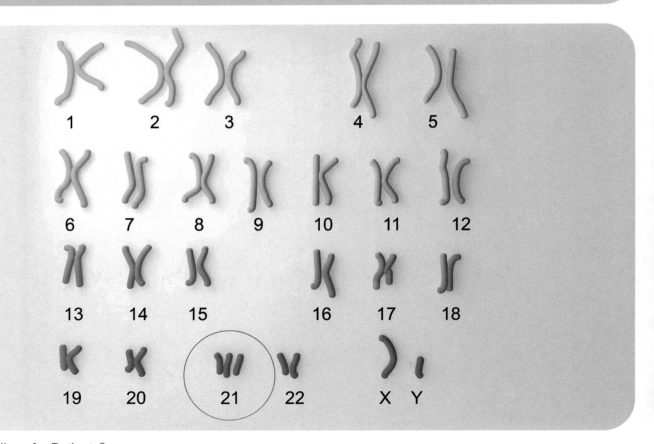

Acute lymphoblastic leukemia (ALL) is the most common cancer diagnosed in children. It is a fast-growing cancer that starts in lymphocytes, a type of white blood cell. Treatment depends on the type of ALL, age at diagnosis, and other factors. Pediatric refers to ALL found in infants, children, and young adults.

Blood

Blood is a tissue. A tissue is a group of cells that work together to perform a function. Blood's function is to move oxygen and nutrients throughout your body and carry away waste. Blood also plays an important role for the immune system.

Blood cells

Your blood contains different types of cells that float in plasma. Plasma is a clear, yellowish fluid made up of mostly water. More than half of your blood is plasma.

There are 3 types of blood cells:

> Red blood cells (erythrocytes)

> White blood cells (leukocytes), which include granulocytes, monocytes, and lymphocytes

> Platelets (thrombocytes)

Blood cells have important jobs. Red blood cells carry oxygen throughout the body. White blood cells fight germs. Platelets help control bleeding.

Blood cells are being replaced in your body all the time. Many have a short lifespan. Some white blood cells live less than one day. Your body makes one million red blood cells every second!

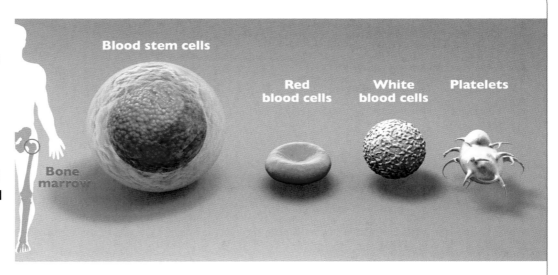

Blood stem cells

Bone marrow contains stem cells. A blood stem cell is an immature cell that can develop into a red blood cell, white blood cell, or platelet.

Blood stem cells

Bone marrow

Red blood cells | White blood cells | Platelets

How blood cells are formed

Bone marrow is the sponge-like tissue in the center of most bones. Inside your bone marrow are early blood-forming cells called blood stem cells (hematopoietic stem cells). All types of blood cells start as blood stem cells. At any given time, bone marrow will have cells in various stages of development, from very immature to almost fully mature.

A blood stem cell has to mature or go through many stages to become a red blood cell, white blood cell, or platelet. With each stage the blood stem cell changes and gets closer to what it is meant to be. After a blood stem cell develops into a red blood cell, white blood cell, or platelet, it is released in your bloodstream as needed.

Blood stem cells can do 2 things:

> Make exact copies of themselves

> Make new cells that have the potential to become blood cells

Blood stem cells can copy themselves or self-renew. These cells are rare. Blood stem cells can also make new cells that are committed to being a certain type of blood cell. These are called progenitor cells or precursor cells. Progenitor cells are much more common than blood stem cells. Progenitor cells can become red blood cells, white blood cells, or platelets.

Blood cell formation

All blood cells start as blood stem cells. A blood stem cell has to mature or go through many stages to become a red blood cell, white blood cell, or platelet. ALL affects the lymphoid progenitor cells, which develop into a type of white blood cell called lymphocytes.

Copyright © 2020 National Comprehensive Cancer Network® (NCCN®). www.nccn.org

blood stem cell

myeloid progenitor cell

lymphoid progenitor cell

myeloblast

lymphoblast

red blood cells

platelets

granulocytes

lymphocytes

There are 2 types of blood progenitor cells:

> Lymphoid

> Myeloid

Lymphoid refers to lymphocyte, a type of white blood cell. Myeloid refers to other types of blood cells in bone marrow. Both lymphoid and myeloid progenitor cells form into blast cells called lymphoblasts or myeloblasts depending on the type. Blasts are committed to becoming a type of white blood cell.

Lymphoid progenitor cells

Lymphoid progenitor cells develop into a type of white blood cell called lymphocytes. Lymphocytes are released from bone marrow into the bloodstream. In ALL, lymphocytes grow out of control in bone marrow. This crowds out blood stems cells and normal red blood cells, platelets, and white blood cells.

Myeloid progenitor cells

Myeloid progenitor cells develop into white blood cells, red blood cells, and platelets. When mature, cells are released from bone marrow into the bloodstream.

Lymphocytes

A lymphocyte is a type of white blood cell found in blood and lymph tissue. Lymph tissue includes lymph vessels and lymph nodes.

There are 3 main types of lymphocytes:

> B lymphocytes or B cells make antibodies. An antibody is a protein.

> T lymphocytes or T cells help kill tumor cells and help control immune responses.

> Natural killer (NK) cells have granules (small particles) with enzymes that can kill tumor cells or cells infected with a virus.

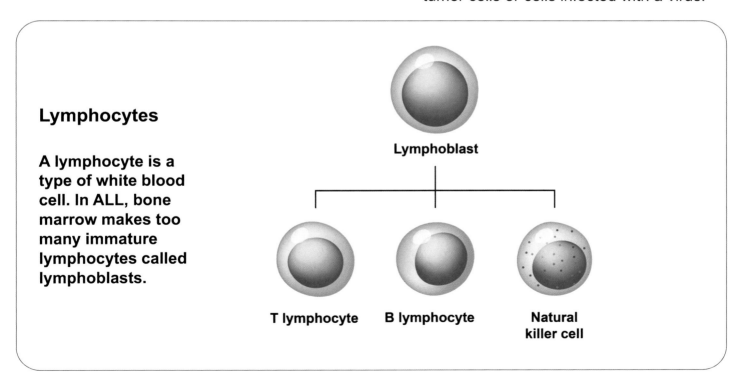

Lymphocytes

A lymphocyte is a type of white blood cell. In ALL, bone marrow makes too many immature lymphocytes called lymphoblasts.

Lymphoblast

T lymphocyte   B lymphocyte   Natural killer cell

ALL most often affects B cells or T cells.

B cell

B cells produce antibodies that are used to attack invading bacteria, viruses, and toxins. The antibody molecules latch on and destroy invading viruses or bacteria.

T cell

T cells are direct fighters of foreign invaders and also produce cytokines, which help activate other parts of the immune system. T cells destroy the body's own cells that have been taken over by viruses or that have become cancerous.

Acute lymphoblastic leukemia

Acute lymphoblastic leukemia (ALL) is a fast-growing blood cancer that starts in disease-fighting lymphocytes of your immune system. In ALL, bone marrow makes too many immature lymphocytes called lymphoblasts. Lymphoblasts can crowd out other blood cells causing blood to not work as it should. Acute leukemias grow faster than chronic leukemias.

To be diagnosed with ALL, 20 percent (20%) or more lymphoblasts must be present in the bone marrow. This means that at least 2 out of every 10 marrow cells are lymphoblasts. In certain cases, a diagnosis of ALL is possible with less than 20% lymphoblasts.

ALL can be found in bone marrow, blood, and organs such as the testicles or the central nervous system.

There are 2 types of pediatric ALL:

> B cell or B-ALL

> T cell or T-ALL

Within each type there are several subtypes, which are based mainly on:

> The type of lymphocyte (most often B cell or T cell) the leukemia cells come from and how mature the cells are. This is known as the immunophenotype of the leukemia.

> If the leukemia cells have certain gene or chromosome changes

B-ALL

B-cell ALL or B-ALL starts in B-cell lymphocytes. B-ALL is more common than T-ALL. Mature B-cell ALL (also called Burkitt leukemia), a rare subtype, is essentially the same as Burkitt lymphoma (a type of non-Hodgkin lymphoma), but is treated differently from B-ALL.

T-ALL

T-cell ALL or T-ALL starts in T-cell lymphocytes. T-ALL can cause an enlarged thymus (a small organ in front of the windpipe), which can sometimes lead to breathing problems.

Abnormal cell changes

Cells in your body contain chromosomes. Chromosomes are long strands of genetic information called DNA (deoxyribonucleic acid). Your DNA uses coded instructions to tell your cells what to do. These instructions are called genes.

Cancer starts when something goes wrong in the DNA of a cell. Abnormal changes in the genes of cancer cells are possible. These abnormal changes are called mutations. Mutations are often found in ALL. ALL can change the DNA in your blood cells.

Types of ALL

ALL is a group of diseases. They are grouped and treated based on gene mutations and other features. Genetic testing is very important to identify the ALL subtype. It is a standard part of testing at diagnosis.

Pediatric ALL

Pediatric refers to ALL found in infants, children, and young adults.

"Pediatric" includes anyone 18 years of age or under, and certain adolescents and young adults (AYAs) over 18 years of age.

AYAs are those 15 to 39 years of age at the time of initial cancer diagnosis. An AYA can be treated in pediatric or adult centers depending on the type of cancer. This book applies to AYAs who are 30 years of age or younger and are being treated at a pediatric cancer center.

For those AYA patients seeking treatment at an adult cancer center, see *NCCN Guidelines for Patients: Acute Lymphoblastic Leukemia*, available at NCCN.org/patientguidelines.

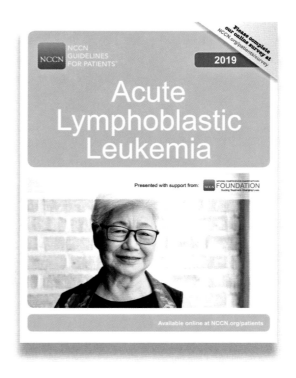

Review

> Acute lymphoblastic leukemia (ALL) is a fast-growing blood cancer. In ALL, bone marrow makes too many immature lymphocytes called lymphoblasts. This makes it hard for blood to do its work.

> To be diagnosed with ALL, 20 percent (20%) or more lymphoblasts must be present in the bone marrow. This means that at least 2 out of every 10 marrow cells are lymphoblasts.

> Pediatric ALL is the most common cancer diagnosed in children. "Pediatric" includes anyone 18 years of age or under, and certain adolescents and young adults (AYAs) over 18 years of age.

> There is more than one type of pediatric ALL. It is based on the type of lymphocyte, genetic mutations, and other features.

Those with pediatric ALL should be treated at experienced pediatric leukemia centers.

2
Testing for ALL

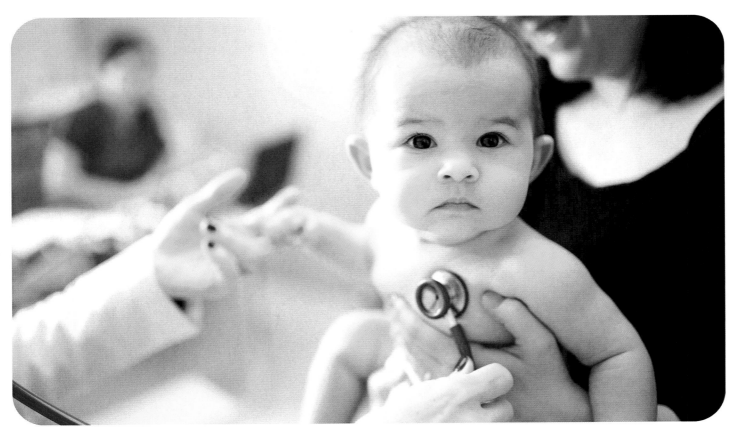

Accurate testing is needed to diagnose and treat pediatric ALL. This chapter presents an overview of possible tests and what to expect.

Test results

Results from blood and tissue tests, imaging studies, and biopsy will determine your treatment plan. It is important you understand what these tests mean. Ask questions and keep copies of your test results. Online patient portals are a great way to access test results.

Whether you are going for a second opinion, test, or office visit, keep these things in mind:

> Both parents can join doctor visits. It is encouraged to ask questions and take notes.

> Get copies of blood tests, imaging results, and reports about the specific type of cancer you have.

> Organize your papers. Create files for insurance forms, medical records, and test results. You can do the same on your computer.

> Keep a list of contact information for everyone on your care team. Add it to your binder or notebook. Hang the list on your fridge or keep it by the phone.

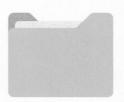

Create a medical binder

A medical binder or notebook is a great way to organize all of your records in one place.

- Make copies of blood tests, imaging results, and reports about your specific type of cancer.

- Choose a binder that meets your needs. Consider a zipper pocket to include a pen, small calendar, and insurance cards.

- Create folders for insurance forms, medical records, and tests results. You can do the same on your computer.

- Use online patient portals to view your test results and other records. Download or print the records to add to your binder.

- Organize your binder in a way that works for you. Add a section for questions and to take notes.

- Bring your medical binder to appointments. You never know when you might need it!

For possible tests, see Guide 1.

Guide 1
Testing for ALL

Medical history and physical exam

Complete blood count (CBC), differential, chemistry profile, liver function tests (LFTs)

Tumor lysis syndrome (TLS) panel: LDH, uric acid, potassium (K), calcium (Ca), phosphorus (Phos)

Disseminated intravascular coagulation (DIC) panel: d-dimer, fibrinogen, prothrombin time (PT), and partial thromboplastin time (PTT)

Pregnancy testing, fertility counseling, and preservation as needed

CT and MRI of head with contrast, if neurologic symptoms

Chest x-ray to rule out mediastinal mass

Whole body PET/CT if lymphoblastic lymphoma suspected

Lumbar puncture (LP) with intrathecal (IT) chemotherapy

Testicular exam, including scrotal ultrasound as needed

Screen for opportunistic infections, as needed

Assessment of left ventricular function (echocardiogram or cardiac nuclear medicine scan) in those who will receive anthracyclines as part of treatment plan

Central venous access device (CVAD) of choice

Consider pharmacogenomic testing for *TPMT, NUDT15*

Consider predisposition syndromes:
- Down syndrome is an important ALL predisposition syndrome.
- For hypodiploid ALL, consider germline *TP53* mutation testing.
- Consider other germline mutation testing.

General health tests

Medical history

A medical history is a record of all health issues and treatments you have had in your life. Be prepared to list any illness or injury and when it happened. Bring a list of old and new medicines and any over-the-counter medicines, herbals, or supplements you take. Tell your doctor about any symptoms you have. A medical history will help determine which treatment is best for you.

Family history

Some cancers and other diseases can run in families. Your doctor will ask about the health history of family members who are blood relatives. This information is called a family history. Ask family members about their health issues like heart disease, cancer, and diabetes, and at what age they were diagnosed.

Leukemia predisposition syndrome

Certain genetic changes, or mutations, can increase a person's chances of developing cancer. These changes, known as hereditary cancer syndromes, can be passed down from parent to child. Your doctor should do a thorough family history and ask if anyone in your family has had leukemia. If there is a concern for a leukemia predisposition syndrome, you might be referred to a genetic counselor or geneticist. Since family members are often bone marrow donors, it is important to rule out leukemia predisposition syndrome.

Physical exam

A physical exam checks the body for signs of disease.

A health care provider may:

> Check your temperature, blood pressure, pulse, and breathing rate

> Weigh you

> Listen to your lungs and heart

> Look in your eyes, ears, nose, and throat

> Feel and apply pressure to parts of your body to see if organs are of normal size, are soft or hard, or cause pain when touched. Tell your doctor if you feel pain.

> Feel for enlarged lymph nodes in your neck, underarm, and groin. Tell the doctor if you have felt any lumps or have any pain.

Doctors should perform a thorough physical exam along with a complete health history.

Testicular exam

ALL can cause swollen testicles. A testicular exam is a complete physical exam of the groin and the genitals, which are the penis, scrotum, and testicles. Your doctor will feel the organs and check for lumps, swelling, shrinking, and other signs of a problem.

Dental exam

The health of your teeth and gums is important. Some treatments can cause dental problems. Therefore, it is important to see a dentist before and during treatment.

Fertility and birth control

Pediatric ALL survivors are at risk for fertility issues. Fertility is the ability to have children. In order to preserve one's fertility, action may be needed before starting cancer treatment. However, this is not always possible.

Those who want to have children in the future should be referred to a fertility specialist to discuss the options. More information can be found in *NCCN Guidelines for Patients: Adolescents and Young Adults with Cancer*, available at NCCN.org/patientguidelines.

> Fertility counseling and/ or preservation options should be presented to everyone with pediatric ALL.

Those with ovaries

Those who can have children will have a pregnancy test before starting treatment. Cancer treatment can hurt the baby if you are or become pregnant during treatment. Therefore, birth control to prevent pregnancy during and after treatment is recommended. Hormonal birth control may not be recommended, so ask your doctor about options.

Those with testicles

Cancer and cancer treatment can damage sperm. Therefore, use contraception (birth control) to prevent pregnancy during and after cancer treatment. If you think you want children in the future, talk to your doctor now. Sperm banking may be an option.

Infertility

Infertility is the complete loss of the ability to have children. The actual risk of infertility is related to your age at time of diagnosis, treatment type(s), treatment dose, and treatment length. Chemotherapy with alkylating agents has a higher risk of infertility. Sometimes, there isn't time for fertility preservation before you start treatment. Talk to your doctor about your concerns.

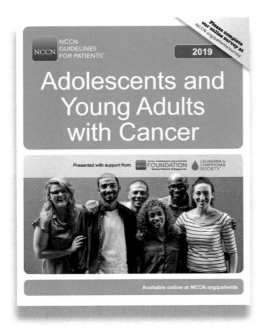

Blood tests

Blood tests check for signs of disease and how well organs are working. They require a sample of blood, which is removed through a needle placed into your vein.

Pregnancy test
Those who can become pregnant will be given a pregnancy test before treatment begins.

Complete blood count
A complete blood count (CBC) measures the levels of red blood cells, white blood cells, and platelets in your blood. Red blood cells carry oxygen throughout your body, white blood cells fight infection, and platelets control bleeding.

Differential
There are 5 types of white blood cells: neutrophils, lymphocytes, monocytes, eosinophils, and basophils. A differential counts the number of each type of white blood cell (WBC). It also checks if the counts are in balance with each other. Your doctor may be able to determine the cause of an abnormal white blood count from this test.

Chemistry profile
A chemistry profile or panel measures different substances in your blood. It provides important information about how well your kidneys and liver are working, among other things.

The liver, bone, and other organs release chemicals in your blood. A chemistry profile measures these levels. This test may be repeated during and after treatment.

> Be prepared to have a lot of blood tests. You might have blood tests as often as every 4 hours during ALL treatment and recovery.

Tumor lysis syndrome panel
Cancer treatment causes cell death. In tumor lysis syndrome (TLS), waste released by dead cells builds up in the body causing kidney damage and severe blood electrolyte disturbances.

Sometimes, TLS is present before treatment starts. If this is the case, allopurinol alone or with rasburicase might be given prior to starting induction chemotherapy.

Induction chemotherapy may cause TLS. It can be life threatening. Drinking lots of water can help.

If you are at risk for TLS, you will have blood tests daily. Changes in creatinine, lactic acid, uric acid, phosphorus (Phos), potassium (K), and calcium (Ca) levels can be sign of TLS.

Creatinine
Creatinine is a waste produced in the muscles. It is filtered out of the blood by the kidneys and tells how well the kidneys are working.

Lactic acid

Lactate dehydrogenase (LDH) or lactic acid dehydrogenase is a protein found in most cells. Dying cells release LDH into blood. Fast-growing cells also release LDH. High levels of LDH can be a sign of ALL.

Uric acid

Uric acid is released by cells when DNA breaks down. It is a normal waste product that dissolves in your blood and is filtered by the kidneys where it leaves the body as urine. Too much uric acid in the body is called hyperuricemia. With ALL, it can be caused by a fast turnover of white blood cells. High uric acid might be a side effect of chemotherapy or radiation therapy.

Liver function tests

Liver function tests (LFTs) look at the health of your liver by measuring chemicals that are made or processed by the liver. Levels that are too high or low signal that the liver is not working well or the bile ducts might be blocked.

Blood clotting tests

Your body stops bleeding by turning blood into a gel-like form. The gel-like blood forms into a solid mass called a blood clot. Clotting is a process or series of events. Proteins, called coagulation factors, are needed for clotting. They are made by the liver. These tests are known together as a coagulation panel or disseminated intravascular coagulation (DIC) panel.

A DIC panel includes:

> D-dimer is present when the body is forming and breaking down blood clots. Prothrombin time (PT) and partial thromboplastin time (PTT) measure how long it takes blood to clot.

> Fibrinogen activity measures how much fibrinogen, a blood protein, is being made by the liver.

An impaired clotting process is common in leukemia. This is called coagulopathy. You may have bleeding and bruises or blood clots. It is standard to screen for clotting problems.

Opportunistic infections

An opportunistic infection can affect those with suppressed immune systems. Drug treatment for ALL can weaken the body's natural defense against infections. You will be monitored for opportunistic infections, as needed.

If not treated early, infections can be fatal. Infections can be caused by viruses, fungus, or bacteria. Antibiotics can treat bacterial infections. Antifungal medicines can treat fungal infections. You may be given antiviral drugs to prevent viral infections.

Spinal fluid tests

Leukemia can travel to the cerebrospinal fluid (CSF) that surrounds the spine or brain. This may cause symptoms. In order to look for leukemia cells in your spinal fluid, a sample must be taken and tested. A lumbar puncture (LP) is a procedure that removes spinal fluid. It is also called a spinal tap.

A lumbar puncture is also used to inject cancer drugs into spinal fluid. This is called intrathecal (IT) chemotherapy. All treatment plans include IT chemotherapy.

A lumbar puncture at diagnosis is used to rule out a central nervous system (CNS) disease.

Tissue tests

A biopsy is the removal of a sample of tissue or group of cells for testing. A diagnosis of ALL is confirmed using either a bone marrow aspirate or bone marrow biopsy.

Bone marrow tests
Leukemia starts in the bone marrow. To diagnose ALL, samples of bone marrow must be removed. Lab results will be used to confirm the disease. Your bone marrow will also be tested to see how well treatment is working.

A hematologist is a doctor who specializes in blood diseases and cancers. A hematopathologist is a doctor who specializes in blood diseases by looking at cells under a microscope. The hematopathologist will study the results of various blood and bone marrow tests and write a report that will be sent to your doctor.

There are 2 types of bone marrow tests that are often done at the same time:

> Bone marrow aspirate

> Bone marrow biopsy

Aspirate and biopsy
Your bone marrow is like a sponge holding liquid. An aspirate takes some of the liquid out of the sponge, and a biopsy takes a piece of the sponge.

The samples are usually taken from the back of the hip bone (pelvis). You will likely lie on your belly or side. Your doctors will first clean and give sedation or numb your skin and outer surface of your bone. For an aspirate, a hollow needle will be pushed through your skin and into the bone. Liquid bone marrow will then be drawn into a syringe. For the biopsy, a wider needle will be used to remove a core sample. You may feel bone pain at your hip for a few days. Your skin may bruise.

Skin punch biopsy
If a predisposition syndrome is suspected, you might have a skin punch biopsy. Genetic testing for leukemia can't be done using blood or saliva. If you tested the blood at diagnosis, you would see the genetic changes of the leukemia. Therefore, a skin punch biopsy is used. In this procedure, a small piece of skin and connective tissue are removed to get DNA that hasn't been altered by ALL. This will be used to see if you have inherited genes that increase your risk of leukemia. Leukemia predisposition syndrome can affect how your body responds to treatment.

Flow cytometry

Flow cytometry involves adding a light-sensitive dye to cells. The dyed cells are passed through a beam of light in a machine. The machine measures the number of cells, things like the size and shape of the cells, and proteins on the surface of thousands of cells.

A blood test can count the number of white blood cells, but it cannot detect the subtle differences between different types of blood cancers. Flow cytometry can detect these subtle differences. It can show if the leukemia cells are mostly myeloid cells or lymphoid cells. This test is important because the cell type may affect which treatment is best for your child.

Imaging tests

Imaging tests take pictures (images) of the inside of your body. These tests are used to look for cancer in organs and areas outside of the blood. A radiologist, an expert in test images, will write a report and send this report to your doctor. Your doctor will discuss the results with you.

Chest x-ray

An x-ray is a type of radiation. In small doses, it is used to make pictures of the inside of the body. A chest x-ray is used to look for a mediastinal mass, which forms in the space between the lungs. This area includes the heart, aorta, esophagus, thymus, trachea, lymph nodes, and nerves.

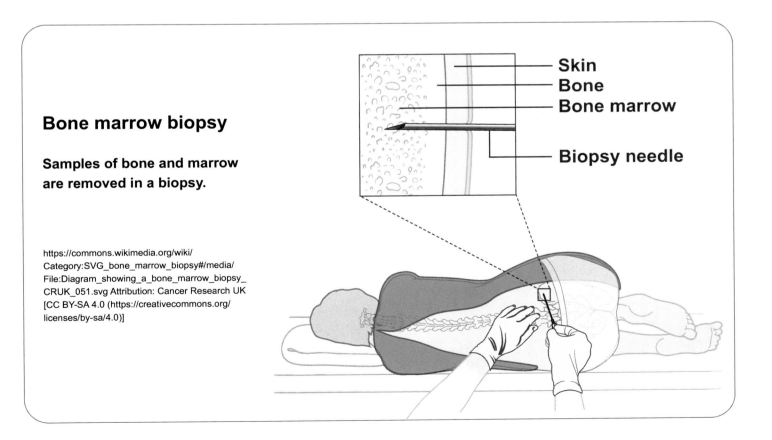

Bone marrow biopsy

Samples of bone and marrow are removed in a biopsy.

Skin
Bone
Bone marrow
Biopsy needle

https://commons.wikimedia.org/wiki/
Category:SVG_bone_marrow_biopsy#/media/
File:Diagram_showing_a_bone_marrow_biopsy_
CRUK_051.svg Attribution: Cancer Research UK
[CC BY-SA 4.0 (https://creativecommons.org/
licenses/by-sa/4.0)]

CT scan

A computed tomography (CT or CAT) scan uses x-rays and computer technology to take pictures of the inside of the body. It takes many x-rays of the same body part from different angles. All the images are combined to make one detailed picture.

A CT scan of your head may be one of the tests to look for cancer. In most cases, contrast will be used. Contrast materials are not dyes, but substances that help certain areas in the body stand out. It is used to make the pictures clearer. The contrast is not permanent and will leave the body in your urine.

Tell your doctors if you have had bad reactions to contrast in the past. This is important. You might be given medicines, such as Benadryl® and prednisone, for an allergy to contrast. Contrast might not be used if you have a serious allergy or if your kidneys aren't working well.

MRI scan

A magnetic resonance imaging (MRI) scan uses radio waves and powerful magnets to take pictures of the inside of the body. It does not use x-rays. Contrast might be used.

PET scan

A positron emission tomography (PET) scan uses a radioactive drug called a tracer. A tracer is a substance injected into a vein to see where it is in the body and if it is using sugar to grow. Cancer cells show up as bright spots on PET scans. Not all bright spots are cancer. It is normal for the brain, heart, kidneys, and bladder to be bright on PET.

Sometimes, PET is combined with CT. This combined test is called a PET/CT scan.

Scrotal ultrasound

A scrotal ultrasound uses sound waves to make images of the scrotum. The scrotum is the pouch of skin at the base of the penis that contains the testicles. The images are recorded on a computer.

Heart tests

Heart or cardiac tests are used to see how well your heart works. These tests might be used to monitor treatment side effects. Your child might be referred to a cardiologist.

Echocardiogram

An echocardiogram (or echo) uses sound waves to make pictures. For this test, small patches will be placed on your chest to track your heartbeat. Next, a wand with gel on its tip will be slid across part of your bare chest. A picture of your beating heart will be seen on a screen. The pictures will be recorded for future viewing.

An echocardiogram is one way of measuring ejection fraction, which is the amount of blood pumped out of the left side of your heart every time it beats. In low ejection fraction, the amount of blood pumping from the left side of the heart is lower than normal.

Cardiac nuclear medicine scan

A nuclear heart scan is an imaging test that uses special cameras and a radioactive substance called a tracer to create pictures of your heart. The tracer is injected into your blood and travels to your heart.

Genetic tests

Genetic tests are used to learn more about your child's type of ALL and to target treatment.

Inside our cells are deoxyribonucleic acid (DNA) molecules. These molecules are tightly packaged into what is called a chromosome. Chromosomes contain most of the genetic information in a cell. Normal human cells contain 23 pairs of chromosomes for a total of 46 chromosomes. Each chromosome contains thousands of genes. Genes tell cells what to do and what to become.

ALL can cause changes in genes and chromosomes in blood cells. Genetic tests look for these changes or abnormalities. Your child may be placed into a risk group based on the types of genetic abnormalities found. There are different types of tests; some are done on molecules or proteins, some on genes, and some on chromosomes. Proteins are written like this: BCR. Genes are written like this: *BCR*.

For a list of some of the genetic abnormalities found in pediatric ALL, see Guide 2.

Karyotype
A karyotype is a picture of chromosomes. It is produced in about a week at a special lab. Doctors look for whether 46 chromosomes or 23 pairs are present. They also look for extra, missing, or abnormal pieces of chromosomes, such as the *BCR-ABL1* gene. Since a karyotype requires growing cells, a sample of bone marrow must be used.

FISH
Fluorescence in situ hybridization (FISH) is a method that involves special dyes called probes that attach to pieces of DNA. For example, the probes attach to the *BCR* gene and the *ABL* gene. The *BCR-ABL1* gene is detected when the colors of the probes overlap by translocation. A translocation is the switching of parts between two chromosomes.

Since this test doesn't need growing cells, it can be performed on either a bone marrow or blood sample. However, FISH can only be used for known changes. It cannot detect all the possible changes found with a karyotype. Sometimes, a bone marrow sample will still be needed to get all of the information your doctor needs to help plan your care.

Doctors can also look for other translocations that are too small to be seen with other methods. Another possible translocation found in ALL is *KMT2A* or t(v;11q23.3).

PCR
A polymerase chain reaction (PCR) is a lab process that can make millions or billions of copies of your DNA (genetic information) in just a few hours, but results can take days. PCR is very sensitive. It can find 1 leukemia cell among more than 100,000 normal cells. This is important when testing not only at diagnosis but also for treatment response or remission.

ALL mutation testing

A sample of your blood or bone marrow will be used to see if ALL cancer cells have any specific mutations. Some mutations can be targeted with specific therapies. This is separate from the genetic testing for mutations that you may have inherited from your parents.

Examples of B-ALL mutations include:

> *ETV6-RUNX1*

Ph-like ALL gene fusions and mutations include:

> Gene fusions involving *ABL1, ABL2, CRLF2, CSF1R, EPOR, JAK2,* or *PDGFRB* (gene fusions)

> Mutations involving *CRLF2, FLT3, IL7R, SH2B3, JAK1, JAK3,* and *JAK2* (in combination with *CRLF2* gene fusions)

Examples of T-ALL mutations include:

> *NOTCH1*

> *TLX1 (HOX11), TLX3 (HOX11L2), LYL1, TAL1,* and *KMT2A*

Guide 2
A list of possible gene or chromosome changes found in ALL

B-ALL with	Hyperdiploidy (leukemia cells with 51 to 67 chromosomes)
	Hypodiploidy (leukemia cells with fewer than 44 chromosomes)
	t(9;22)(q34;q11.2) translocation that results in *BCR-ABL1*
	t(v;11q23.3) translocation that results in *KMT2A rearranged*
	t(12;21)(p13;q22) translocation that results in *ETV6-RUNX1*
	t(1;19)(q23;p13.3) translocation that results in *TCF3-PBX1*
	t(5;14)(q31.1;q32.1) translocation that results in *IL3-IGH*
	B-lymphoblastic leukemia/lymphoma with translocations involving tyrosine kinases or cytokine receptors (also known as *BCR-ABL1*–like ALL or Ph-like ALL)
	B-lymphoblastic leukemia/lymphoma with intrachromosomal amplification (too many copies) of a portion of chromosome 21 (*iAMP21*)
T-ALL with	T-ALL is characterized by activating mutations of *NOTCH1*, and rearrangements of transcription factors *TLX1 (HOX11), TLX3 (HOX11L2), LYL1, TAL1,* and *KMT2A.*
	Early T-cell precursor (ETP-ALL) lymphoblastic leukemia and natural killer (NK) cell lymphoblastic leukemia/lymphoma

Philadelphia chromosome

All cells in our body contain genetic information organized in chromosomes. A cell must make a copy of its chromosomes before dividing into two cells. Sometimes, there are mistakes in the copies. One type of mistake is when parts of two chromosomes break off and switch with each other. This is called a translocation. It can result in a fusion gene. There are a few different translocations that might be found in pediatric ALL. One is the Philadelphia chromosome (Ph).

In the Philadelphia chromosome, a piece of chromosome 9 and a piece of chromosome 22 break off and trade places with each other. These pieces then fuse together on chromosome 22. This new, abnormal chromosome 22 is referred to as the Philadelphia chromosome. You might see it written as Ph-positive (Ph+).

The piece of chromosome 9 is a gene called *ABL*. The piece of chromosome 22 is a gene called *BCR*. When these genes fuse together on chromosome 22, the *BCR-ABL1* gene is formed. *BCR-ABL1* is a fusion gene. It is not found in normal blood cells. It is not passed down from parents to children.

BCR-ABL1 makes a new protein that leads to uncontrolled cell growth. Treatment for Ph+ ALL aims to stop the activity of the *BCR-ABL* fusion protein. Genes are written like this: *BCR-ABL*. Proteins are written like this: BCR-ABL.

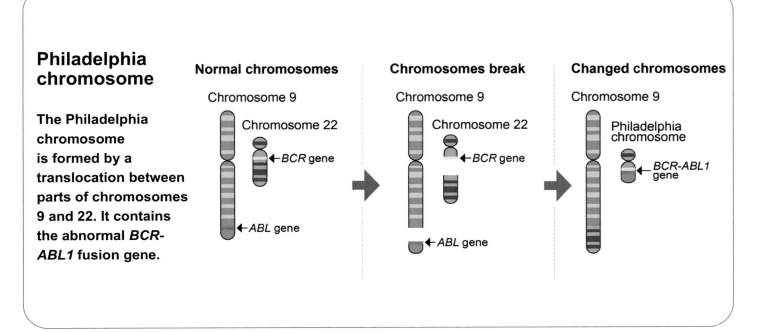

Philadelphia chromosome

The Philadelphia chromosome is formed by a translocation between parts of chromosomes 9 and 22. It contains the abnormal *BCR-ABL1* fusion gene.

Normal chromosomes
Chromosome 9
Chromosome 22
← *BCR* gene
← *ABL* gene

Chromosomes break
Chromosome 9
Chromosome 22
← *BCR* gene
← *ABL* gene

Changed chromosomes
Chromosome 9
Philadelphia chromosome
← *BCR-ABL1* gene

Immunophenotyping

Immunophenotyping (said immuno-feeno-typing) uses antibodies to detect the presence or absence of white blood cell antigens. These antigens are proteins that can be found on the surface of or inside white blood cells. They are called markers or biomarkers. Certain biomarkers are targeted in ALL treatment.

Immunophenotyping is done using flow cytometry. It is used to pinpoint the type of ALL.

Based on immunophenotype, ALL can be placed into 2 general groups:

> B-cell ALL

> T-cell ALL

B-ALL
B-ALL is the most common type of pediatric ALL. It starts in immature cells (lymphoblasts) that would normally develop into B-lymphocytes. Subtypes include early precursor B-cell (early pre–B-cell) and pre–B-cell. Mature B-cell ALL (Burkitt lymphoma) is a rare subtype.

T-ALL
T-ALL starts in lymphoblasts that would normally develop into T-cell lymphocytes. This type is less common, and it occurs more often in adolescent boys. A protein called CD3 is typically found in T-ALL. Others may be present. Early T-cell precursor (ETP-ALL) is a distinct subtype of T-ALL.

Pharmacogenomic testing

Pharmacogenomics (said farma-co-gee-nome-icks) is the study of how genes affect a person's response to drugs. How well your body absorbs (metabolizes) drugs is an important factor in treatment. Not everyone receives the same dose. Your age, weight, and other factors play a role in the dose you receive. Therefore, you will have a test to find the best starting dose for you.

This test looks for genes that help to guide dosing decisions.

Two examples are as follows:

> Thiopurine methyltransferase (TPMT)

> Nudix hydrolase 15 (NUDT15)

Based on the results of the test, your child might start certain types of chemotherapy at a lower dose. This gives the body time to adjust and for the treatment team time to watch for myelosuppression. In myelosuppression, bone marrow activity is decreased, resulting in fewer red blood cells, white blood cells, and platelets. This is supposed to happen with certain chemotherapies.

Risk groups

There are different levels of risk. Your child might be placed into one of the following risk groups: low risk (LR), standard risk (SR), high risk (HR), and very high risk (VHR).

Risk factors include:

- Predisposition syndrome
- Down syndrome
- Hypodiploidy or hyperdiploidy
- Age
- White blood cell (WBC) count at diagnosis
- Gene or chromosome mutations

Risk groups and treatment planning are based on testing lymphoblasts in bone marrow or blood for specific genetic abnormalities.

Tests performed include:

- Karyotype
- Fluorescence in situ hybridization (FISH)
- Reverse transcriptase-polymerase chain reaction (RT-PCR) of *BCR-ABL1* in B-ALL
- If *BCR-ABL1* negative, then possible tests for gene fusions and mutations associated with *BCR-ABL1*-like (Ph-like) ALL

How ALL responds to treatment and if minimal residual disease remains after treatment also play a role.

Predisposition syndrome
Some hereditary cancer syndromes can be passed down from parent to child. A family history of leukemia can affect treatment.

Down syndrome
In Down syndrome, there is an extra chromosome 21. Instead of two chromosomes, there are three. There are challenges treating those with Down syndrome.

Hypodiploidy
In hypodiploidy, leukemia cells have fewer than 44 chromosomes. Normal cells have 46 chromosomes.

Hyperdiploidy
In hyperdiploidy, leukemia cells have more than 50 chromosomes. Normal cells have 46 chromosomes.

Age
ALL tends to be more aggressive in infants and those 10 years of age and over. Infants are those under the age of 12 months (1 year).

WBC
A WBC greater than 50,000/μL at initial diagnosis is considered high risk.

B-ALL genetic risk groups
Your child will be placed into an initial risk group based on the genetic features (mutations) found in the leukemia cells. Some genetic mutations respond better to treatment. Unfavorable risk features are more of a challenge to treat. At certain treatment milestones risk group might be re-assessed by considering response to treatment.

Some of the genetic mutations for B-ALL are shown in Guide 3.

Get to know your care team and let them get to know you.

Guide 3
Genetic risk groups for B-ALL

Favorable risk features	High hyperdiploidy (leukemia cells have 51 to 67 chromosomes) • Trisomy of chromosomes 4, 10, and 17 are among trisomies that have the most favorable outcome
	Cryptic t(12;21)(p13;q22): *ETV6-RUNX1* fusion
Unfavorable risk features	Hypodiploidy (leukemia cells have less than 44 chromosomes)
	KMT2Ar (t[4;11] or others)
	t(9;22)(q34;q11.2): *BCR-ABL1*
	BCR-ABL1-like (Ph-like) ALL • JAK-STAT (*CRLF2r, EPORr, JAK1/2/3r, TYK2r*, mutations of *SH2B3, IL7R, JAK1/2/3*) • ABL class (rearrangements of *ABL1, ABL2, PDGFRA, PDGFRB, FGFR*) • Other (*NTRKr, FLT3r, LYNr, PTL2Br*)
	t(17;19): *TCF3-HLF* fusion
	Intrachromosomal amplification of chromosome 21 (*iAMP21*)
	Alterations of *IKZF1*

HLA typing

A human leukocyte antigen (HLA) is a protein found on the surface of most cells. It plays an important role in your body's immune response. HLAs are unique to each person. They mark your body's cells. Your body detects these markers to tell which cells are yours. In other words, all your cells have the same set of HLAs. Each person's set of HLAs is called the HLA type or tissue type.

HLA typing is a test that detects a person's HLA type. This test is done before a donor blood stem cell transplant. Your proteins will be compared to the donor's white blood cells to see how many proteins are the same in order to find the best match. A very good match is needed for a transplant to be a treatment option. Otherwise, your body will reject the donor cells or the donor cells will react against your body. Blood samples from you and your blood relatives will be tested first.

Review

> Results from blood and tissue tests, imaging studies, and biopsy will determine the treatment plan.

> A biopsy is the removal of a sample of tissue or group of cells for testing. A diagnosis of ALL is confirmed using either a bone marrow aspirate or bone marrow biopsy.

> Immunophenotyping is used to pinpoint the type of pediatric ALL.

> Your child may might be placed into a risk group before starting treatment. Risk might be reassessed between stages of treatment.

> Factors that can affect treatment include age, white blood cell count at diagnosis, predisposition syndrome, Down syndrome, and gene or chromosome mutations.

> Cancer treatment can affect fertility.

> Blood tests check for signs of disease, how well organs are working, and treatment results. Blood clotting tests will also be done.

> Imaging tests are used to look for sites of infection, bleeding, and leukemia that might have spread outside the bloodstream.

> Heart or cardiac tests are used to see how well your heart works. These tests might be used to monitor treatment side effects.

> Leukemia can travel to the cerebrospinal fluid (CSF) that surrounds the spine or brain. It can also travel to sites outside of the blood such as the testicles.

3
Treating pediatric ALL

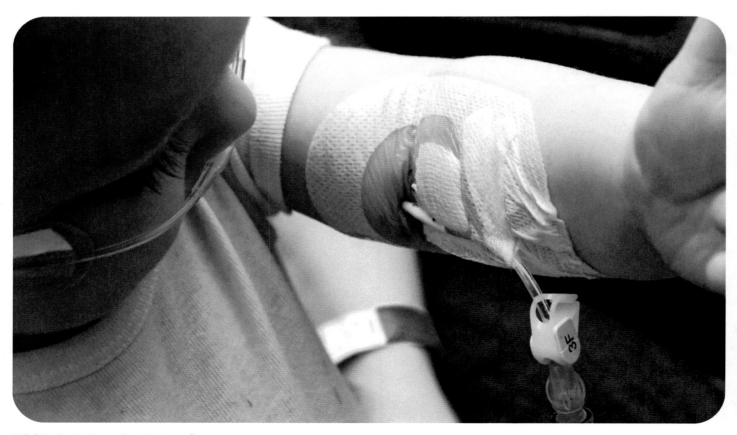

There is more than one treatment for pediatric ALL. This chapter presents an overview of the types of treatment and what to expect. Not everyone will receive the same treatment.

Overview

Chemotherapy is the backbone of pediatric ALL treatment and is often combined with other drug therapies. Chemotherapy is a type of systemic drug therapy that kills fast-growing cells throughout the body, including cancer cells and normal cells.

Chemotherapy, fluids, and blood products might be given through:

> Central venous access device (CVAD)

> Peripheral intravenous (PIV) line

Your child will likely get either a catheter or a port to deliver chemotherapy and other treatments. A catheter is a thin, long tube that is often placed in the chest. This goes into a large vein and stays there until treatment is complete. A port is a small, round disc that is usually placed in the chest. Ask which option is best for your child based on the treatment they will be receiving.

CVAD
A central venous access device (CVAD) and central venous catheter (CVC or central line) are devices inserted into the body through a vein. This makes it easier to give fluids, blood products, medicine, and other therapies directly into the bloodstream. The device may be a catheter (examples include Hickman and Broviac) or port (port-a-cath). The device will be inserted during a minor surgery and remain in your body until treatment is complete. Once the CVAD is removed, the skin will heal.

CVADs can be inserted into a vein in the neck (jugular) or under the collarbone (subclavian). It can be inserted into one of the peripheral veins of the upper arm. While generally safe, there are risks for infection and blood clots.

PICC
A peripherally inserted central catheter (PICC or PICC line) is a long, thin tube that's inserted through a vein in your arm and passed through to the larger veins near your heart.

PIV
A peripheral intravenous line (PIV) is a small, short plastic catheter that is placed through the skin into a vein, usually in the hand, elbow, or foot. A PIV can be used to give fluids, medicines, and certain chemotherapies.

Children will experience new and unusual sensations. They will take cues from you. If you are anxious or worried, your child will likely feel the same.

Chemotherapy

Children and young adults can tolerate higher doses than adults. However, with higher doses there are side effects. Your child will be monitored throughout treatment for side effects or other unwanted (adverse) reactions.

Chemotherapy can be given as follows:

> **Oral (PO)** – taken by mouth either as a liquid or pill

> **Subcutaneous (SQ) -** given under the skin

> **Intramuscular (IM)** – uses a needle to inject medicine in the muscle of the arm or leg (like the flu shot)

> **IV (intravenous) infusion** – chemotherapy administered through a vein using IV push, gravity infusion, or infusion pump. In an IV push, a drug is injected quickly over a few minutes. With a gravity infusion, medicine is put into a bag that hangs on a pole, and the pressure of gravity delivers the medicine into the IV line at a safe and steady rate. In an IV infusion, chemotherapy flows through a tube attached to the catheter. The flow may be controlled by a machine called an IV pump.

> **Intrathecal (IT)** – chemotherapy administered into the spinal fluid. In addition to other forms of chemotherapy, all children get chemotherapy injected into the cerebrospinal fluid (CSF) to kill any leukemia cells that might have spread to the brain and spinal cord. This treatment is given through a lumbar puncture (spinal tap).

Types of chemotherapy

Chemotherapies used to treat ALL disrupt the life cycle of cancer cells. There are many types of chemotherapy used to treat ALL. Often chemotherapies are combined. This is called multi-agent chemotherapy.

Some types of chemotherapies used to treat pediatric ALL are described next.

Alkylating agents

Alkylating agents damage DNA by adding a chemical to it. This group of drugs includes cyclophosphamide.

Anthracyclines

Anthracyclines damage and disrupt the making of DNA causing cell death of both cancerous and non-cancerous cells.

Examples of anthracyclines include:

> Daunorubicin (Cerubidine®)

> Idarubicin (Idamycin PFS®)

> Doxorubicin (Adriamycin)

Antimetabolites

Antimetabolites prevent the "building blocks" of DNA from being used.

Examples of antimetabolites include:

> Cytarabine (Cytosar-U®)

> Fludarabine (Fludara®)

> Clofarabine (Clolar®)

> Methotrexate

> 6-MP (6-mercaptopurine)

> Thioguanine (Tabloid®)

> Nelarabine (Arranon®)

> Tell your doctor about any medications, vitamins, over-the-counter drugs, herbals, or supplements you are taking.

Steroids

Steroid is the short name for corticosteroid. Steroids are man-made versions of hormones made by the adrenal glands. The adrenal glands are small structures found near the kidneys, which help regulate blood pressure and reduce inflammation.

Steroids also are toxic to lymphoid cells and are an important part of pediatric ALL chemotherapy. Steroids can cause short-term and long-term side effects. Corticosteroids are not the same as the steroids used by some athletes.

Steroids include:

> Dexamethasone

> Prednisone

> Hydrocortisone

Enzyme therapy
All cells in the body need the amino acid asparagine to survive. Normal white blood cells can make their own asparagine, but cancerous white blood cells cannot. Asparaginase is an enzyme that speeds up the breakdown of asparagine in the blood. This lowers the level of asparagine in the body. Without asparagine, leukemia cells die.

Pegaspargase (Oncaspar®), calaspargase (Asparlas™), or asparaginase derived from *Erwinia chrysanthemi* (Erwinaze® or ERW) are some types of enzyme therapy used in chemotherapy treatment.

Plant alkaloids
Plant alkaloids are made from plants. Plant alkaloids are cell-cycle specific. This means they attack the cells during various phases of division. Vincristine (also known as Oncovin® or Vincasar PFS®) belongs in a class of drugs called vinca alkaloids. It is also a microtubule inhibitor. Microtubule inhibitors stop a cell from dividing into two cells.

Targeted therapy

Targeted therapy is a form of systemic therapy that works throughout your body. It is a drug therapy that focuses on specific or unique features of cancer cells.

Targeted therapies seek out how cancer cells grow, divide, and move in the body. These drugs stop the action of molecules that help cancer cells grow and/or survive.

Tyrosine kinase inhibitor

A tyrosine kinase inhibitor (TKI) is a type of targeted therapy that blocks the signals that cause cancer to grow and spread. TKIs might be used alone or in combination with other systemic therapies like chemotherapy.

Tyrosine kinases are proteins in cells that are important for many cell functions. The protein made by the *BCR-ABL1* gene is a tyrosine kinase. It moves or transfers chemicals, called phosphates, from one molecule to another. TKIs block this transfer, which stops cell growth.

Each TKI works in a slightly different way. You might not be given a certain TKI if you have a health condition, such as lung or heart issues.

TKIs used to treat ALL
Below are some of the TKIs used to treat pediatric ALL:

> Dasatinib (Sprycel®)

> Imatinib (Gleevec®)

> Ruxolitinib (Jakafi®)

Warnings!

You might be asked to stop taking or avoid certain herbal supplements when on a TKI, chemotherapy, or steroid. Some supplements can affect the ability of a drug to do its job. This is called a drug interaction. It is critical to speak with your care team about any supplements you may be taking.

These include:

> Turmeric

> Gingko biloba

> Green tea extract

> St. John's Wort

Even certain medicines can affect the ability of a TKI to do its job. Antacids, heart medicine, and antidepressants are just some of the medicines that might interact with a targeted therapy. This is why it is important to tell your doctor about any medications, vitamins, over-the-counter (OTC) drugs, herbals, or supplements you are taking. **Bring a list with you to every visit.**

Immunotherapy

Immunotherapy is a targeted therapy that increases the activity of your immune system. By doing so, it improves your body's ability to find and destroy cancer cells. Immunotherapy can be given alone or with other types of treatment.

Monoclonal antibody therapy

Antibody therapy uses antibodies to help the body fight cancer, infection, or other diseases. Antibodies are proteins made by the immune system that bind to specific markers on cells or tissues. Monoclonal antibodies are a type of antibody made in the lab. In cancer treatment, monoclonal antibodies may kill cancer cells directly, they may block development of tumor blood vessels, or they may help the immune system kill cancer cells.

> Blinatumomab (Blincyto®) allows normal T cells to attack cancerous B cells by bringing them close together. Blinatumomab may cause severe, life-threatening, or fatal reactions.

> Inotuzumab ozogamicin (Besponsa™) binds to CD22 on leukemia cells then releases a toxic agent once it's inside the cells. Inotuzumab ozogamicin is not FDA approved for children and can cause fatal and life-threatening reactions.

CD19-targeting CAR T-cell therapy

CD19-directed genetically modified autologous T-cell immunotherapy is made from your own T cells. T cells will be removed from your body, and in the lab, a CAR (chimeric antigen receptor) will be added to them. This programs the T cells to find leukemia cells. The programmed T cells will be infused back into your body to find and kill cancer cells. This treatment is not for everyone. There can be severe and sometimes life-threatening reactions.

Tisagenlecleucel (Kymriah™) is a type of CD19-targeting CAR T-cell therapy.

More information on CAR T-cell therapy can be found in *NCCN Guidelines for Patients: Immunotherapy Side Effects*, available at NCCN.org/patientguidelines.

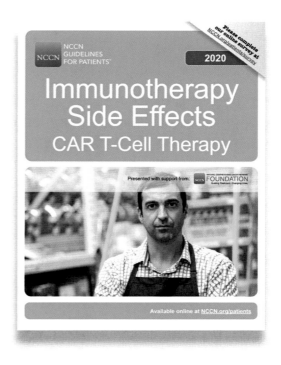

Radiation therapy

Radiation therapy (RT) uses high-energy radiation from x-rays, gamma rays, protons, and other sources to kill cancer cells and shrink tumors. It is given over a certain period of time. Radiation therapy can be given alone or with certain systemic therapies. It may be used as supportive care to help ease pain or discomfort caused by cancer.

> Those with leukemia in the central nervous system at diagnosis may receive radiation to the brain area.

> Those with testicular disease at diagnosis that remains after induction therapy may receive radiation to the testes.

Cranial irradiation

In cranial irradiation, the areas of the brain targeted for ALL treatment are different from areas targeted for brain metastases of solid tumors.

Total body irradiation

Total body irradiation (TBI) is radiation of the whole body given before bone marrow transplant.

Bone marrow transplant

A bone marrow transplant (BMT) replaces bone marrow stem cells. You might hear it called a hematopoietic stem cell transplant (HSCT) or stem cell transplant (SCT). This book will refer to it as SCT.

There are 2 types of SCTs:

> Autologous – stem cells come from you

> Allogeneic – stem cells come from a donor that may or may not be related to you

Only an allogeneic SCT is used as a treatment option for pediatric ALL. An SCT depends upon donor availability and your child's health at the time of potential SCT. The steps of an allogeneic SCT are described next.

Conditioning

Before an SCT, treatment is needed to destroy bone marrow cells. This is called conditioning and it creates room for the healthy donor stem cells. It also weakens the immune system so your body won't kill the transplanted cells.

There are 2 main types of conditioning:

> **High-dose conditioning** consists of high doses of strong chemotherapy. High-dose conditioning can cause life-threatening side effects. Also, not everybody can tolerate it.

> **Reduced-intensity conditioning** consists of low doses of strong chemotherapy. It may also consist of low-intensity drugs. Reduced-intensity conditioning may be used for people who are older or less healthy overall. However, the chance for a cancer relapse can be greater compared to high-dose conditioning.

Radiation therapy may also be given as part of conditioning treatment.

Transplanting stem cells

After conditioning, you will receive the healthy stem cells through a transfusion. A transfusion is a slow injection of blood products into a vein. This can take several hours. The transplanted stem cells will travel to your bone marrow and grow. New, healthy blood cells will form. This is called engraftment. It usually takes about 2 to 4 weeks.

Until then, you will have little or no immune defense. You may need to stay in a very clean room at the hospital or be given antibiotics to prevent or treat infection. Transfusions are also possible. A red blood cell transfusion is used to prevent bleeding and to treat anemia (below normal red blood cell count). A platelet transfusion is used to treat a low platelet count or bleeding. While waiting for the cells to engraft, you will likely feel tired and weak.

Possible side effects

Every treatment has side effects. Your child will be monitored for infections, disease relapse, and graft-versus-host disease (GVHD). In GVHD, the donor cells attack your normal, healthy tissue. There are treatments for GVHD. Ask about the possible side effects or complications of SCT and how this might affect your child's quality of life.

> A stem cell transplant (SCT) depends upon donor availability and your child's health at the time of potential SCT.

Clinical trials

A clinical trial is a type of research study that tests new methods of screening, prevention, diagnosis, or treatment of a disease.

Clinical trials have 4 phases.

> **Phase I trials** aim to find the safest and best dose of a new drug. Another aim is to find the best way to give the drug with the fewest side effects.

> **Phase II trials** assess if a drug works for a specific type of cancer.

> **Phase III trials** compare a new drug to a standard treatment.

> **Phase IV trials** evaluate a drug's long-term safety and effectiveness after it has been approved.

Those in a clinical trial often are alike in terms of their cancer type or stage and general health. This helps ensure that any change is a result of the treatment and not due to differences between participants.

If you decide to join a clinical trial, you will need to review and sign an informed consent form. This form describes the study in detail, including the risks and benefits. Even after you sign a consent form, you can stop taking part in a clinical trial at any time.

Ask your treatment team if there is an open clinical trial that you can join. Discuss the risks and benefits of joining a clinical trial with your care team. Together, decide if a clinical trial is right for you.

Finding a clinical trial

Enrollment in a clinical trial is encouraged when it is the best option for you.

- To find clinical trials online at NCCN Cancer Centers, go to NCCN.org/clinical_trials/member_institutions.aspx

- To search the National Institutes of Health (NIH) database for clinical trials in the United States and around the world, go to ClinicalTrials.gov

- To find clinical trials supported by the National Cancer Institute (NCI), go to cancer.gov/about-cancer/treatment/clinical-trials/search

Ask your cancer team for help finding a clinical trial. You may also get help from NCI's Cancer Information Service (CIS). Call 1.800.4.CANCER (1.800.422.6237) or go to cancer.gov/contact

Supportive care

Supportive care will be specific to your child's needs. Supportive care is health care that relieves symptoms caused by cancer or its treatment and improves quality of life. It might include pain relief (palliative care), emotional or spiritual support, financial aid, or family counseling. Supportive care and palliative care are often used interchangeably. Supportive care is always given.

Some potential side effects and procedures are described next.

Side effects

All cancer treatments can cause unwanted health issues called side effects. Side effects depend on many factors. These factors include the drug type and dose, length of treatment, and the person. Some side effects may be harmful to your health. Others may just be unpleasant. Pediatric ALL treatment can cause a number of side effects. Some are very serious.

Late effects

Late effects are side effects that occur months or years after a disease is diagnosed or after treatment has ended. Late effects may be caused by cancer or cancer treatment. They may include physical, mental, and social problems, and second cancers. The sooner late effects are treated the better. Ask your care team about what late effects could occur. This will help you know what to look for.

Blood clots

Cancer treatment can cause blood clots to form. This can block blood flow and oxygen in the body. Blood clots can break loose and travel to other parts of the body causing stroke or other problems.

Cytokine release syndrome

Cytokine release syndrome (CRS) is a condition that may occur after treatment with some types of immunotherapy, such as monoclonal antibodies and CAR-T cells. It is caused by a large, rapid release of cytokines from immune cells affected by the immunotherapy. Signs and symptoms of CRS include fever, muscle aches, nausea, headache, rash, fast heartbeat, low blood pressure, and trouble breathing.

Dialysis

There are different types of dialysis. Dialysis is the process of filtering blood when the kidneys are unable. Hemodialysis and hemofiltration remove waste and water by circulating blood outside the body through an external filter.

Distress

Distress is an unpleasant experience of a mental, physical, social, or spiritual nature. It can affect how you feel, think, and act. Distress might include feelings of sadness, fear, helplessness, worry, anger, and guilt. You may also experience depression, anxiety, and sleeping problems. Keep in mind, children show signs of distress differently than adults.

For more information, read *NCCN Guidelines for Patients: Distress During Cancer Care*, available at NCCN.org/patientguidelines.

High blood pressure

High blood pressure (HBP or hypertension) occurs when the force of blood flowing through your blood vessels is consistently too high. This can cause headaches and vision problems. If left untreated, HPB can cause heart problems and stroke. Steroids can cause HBP. Medicine might be used to control HBP.

High blood sugar

One possible side effect of steroids is high blood sugar or hyperglycemia. Glucose (sugar found in the blood) will be measured. Insulin might be needed to control high blood sugar.

Hyperleukocytosis

Hyperleukocytosis (leukostasis) is an extremely high lymphoblast count. It occurs most often in those with a very high white blood cell count (usually more than 200 × 10⁹/L), T-cell immunophenotype, and *BCR-ABL1*, and in infants with *KMT2A* rearrangement.

Hypersensitivity, allergy, and anaphylaxis

Certain treatments can cause an unwanted reaction. Hypersensitivity is an exaggerated response by the immune system to a drug or other substance. This can include hives, skin welts, and trouble breathing. An allergy is an immune reaction to a substance that normally is harmless or would not cause an immune response in most people. An allergic response may cause harmful symptoms such as itching or inflammation (swelling). Anaphylaxis or anaphylactic shock is a severe and possible life-threatening allergic reaction.

Infection

Your child will be monitored for signs of infection. Fever can be a sign of infection. Patients are at a higher risk for infection when they have neutropenia. Neutropenia is an abnormally low number of neutrophils (a type of white blood cell) in the blood. Antibiotics might be used to treat infection. Blood or urine may be tested when infection is suspected.

Leukapheresis

In leukapheresis, you will be connected to a machine called a centrifuge. The centrifuge separates white blood cells (leukocytes) from other blood cells. Once the excess leukocytes are removed, the blood is returned to your body. It is also called leukocytapheresis.

Nausea and vomiting

Nausea and vomiting are a common side effect of treatment. You will be given medicine to prevent nausea and vomiting.

For more information, read the *NCCN Guidelines for Patients: Nausea and Vomiting*, available at NCCN.org/patientguidelines.

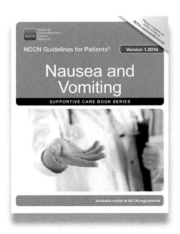

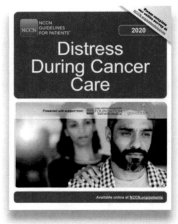

Neurocognitive effects

Some treatments can damage the nervous system (neurotoxicity) causing problems with concentration and memory. Survivors are at risk for neurotoxicity and might be recommended for neuropsychological testing. Neuropsychology looks at how the health of your brain affects your thinking and behavior. Neuropsychological testing can identify your limits and doctors can create a plan to help with these limits.

Neurotoxicity

If ALL treatment includes methotrexate, then you will be monitored for methotrexate neurotoxicity (MTX). Neurotoxicity, such as seizures and confusion, can be seen with immunotherapy, as well.

Neuropathy

Neuropathy is a nerve problem that causes pain, numbness, tingling, swelling, or muscle weakness in different parts of the body. It usually begins in the hands or feet and gets worse over time. Neuropathy may be caused by cancer or cancer treatment.

Organ issues

Treatment might cause your kidneys, liver, heart, and pancreas to not to work as well as they should.

Osteonecrosis

Osteonecrosis, or avascular necrosis, is death of bone tissue due to lack of blood supply. It is a possible side effect of steroids and most often affects weight-bearing joints, such as the hip and/or knee.

Pain

Tell your care team about any pain or discomfort. Your child might meet with a pediatric pain or palliative care specialist to manage pain. Bone pain and vincristine-associated neuropathic pain are common in ALL.

Pneumonia

Pneumocystis pneumonia is a serious infection caused by the fungus *Pneumocystis jirovecii*. Since those with ALL are at high risk, medicine will be given throughout treatment to prevent this type of pneumonia.

Survivorship

A survivor is someone with a history of cancer. A person is a cancer survivor from the time of diagnosis until end of life. When treatment leads to remission (or no evidence of disease), you will need follow-up or survivorship care. During survivorship care your child will still have a care team, but it will look different. Your child will need support. Seek out peer support groups, whether online or in-person.

Therapy-related toxicity

Many of the drug therapies used to treat pediatric ALL can be harmful to the body. Your child will be closely monitored for therapy-related toxicity.

Transfusions

Blood transfusions are common during ALL treatment. A transfusion is a slow injection of blood products such as red blood cells or platelets into a vein. Over time, the body may begin to reject blood transfusions.

Trouble eating

Sometimes side effects from surgery, cancer, or its treatment might cause you to feel not hungry or sick to your stomach (nauseated). You might have a sore mouth. Healthy eating is important during treatment. It includes eating a balanced diet, eating the right amount of food, and drinking enough fluids. A registered dietitian who is an expert in nutrition and food can help. Speak to your care team if you have trouble eating or maintaining weight.

Tumor lysis syndrome

Tumor lysis syndrome (TLS) causes an imbalance of substances in blood. There are different treatments for TLS. Treatment depends on what substances are out of balance and how well your kidneys are working. Sometimes, TLS can cause too much potassium in your blood. Treatment might include hemodialysis or hemofiltration. A machine will filter your blood.

Weight gain

Weight gain is one side effect of high-dose steroids. This can be uncomfortable and cause distress. It is important to maintain muscle mass. Try to find an activity you enjoy. Ask your care team what can be done to help manage weight gain.

Review

> Chemotherapy kills fast-growing cells throughout the body, including cancer cells and normal cells.

> Steroids are part of ALL regimens.

> Targeted therapy focuses on specific or unique features of cancer cells.

> Immunotherapy increases the activity of your immune system.

> A bone marrow transplant (BMT) replaces damaged bone marrow stem cells with healthy stem cells. You might hear it called a hematopoietic stem cell transplant (HSCT) or stem cell transplant (SCT).

> Clinical trials study how safe and helpful tests and treatments are for people. Many ALL treatment regimens are the result of clinical trials.

> Supportive care is health care that relieves symptoms caused by cancer or its treatment and improves quality of life. Supportive care is always given.

> All cancer treatments can cause unwanted health issues called side effects. You will be monitored for side effects, infection, and other treatment-related issues.

> Some side effects, called late effects, may take years to appear. Risk for late effects will depend on the type(s) of cancer treatment you had, and the dose and the length of time you were treated. It is important to go to follow-up appointments.

4
Treatment phases

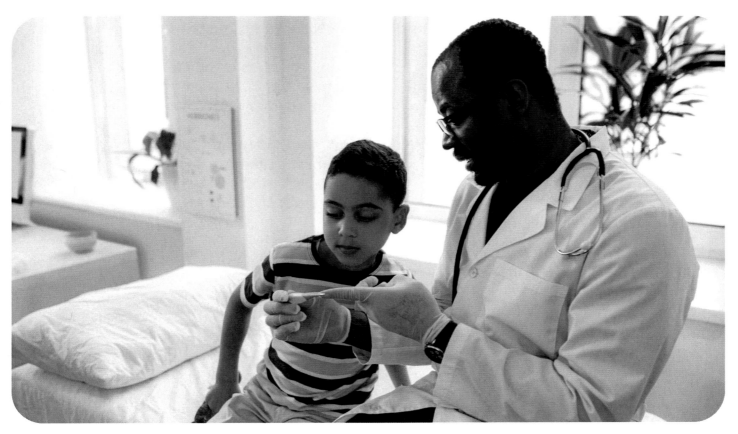

The goal of treatment is a complete response or complete remission. Treatment will be in phases. The three phases of treatment are induction, consolidation, and maintenance.

Types of response

There are different types of treatment response. When there are no signs of cancer, it is called a complete response (CR) or complete remission. This does not always mean that ALL has been cured. Remission can be short-term (temporary) or long-lasting (permanent).

A diagnosis of ALL is based on the presence of 20 percent (20%) or more lymphoblasts in the bone marrow. This means that at least 2 out of every 10 marrow cells are lymphoblasts. However, in some cases a diagnosis of ALL is possible with less than 20% blasts. Treatment aims to reduce the number of blasts.

In complete response all of the following are true:

> Absolute neutrophil count (ANC) is more than 1,000/µL

> Platelet count is more than 100,000/µL

> No lymphoblasts are found in blood

> Less than 5% blasts are found in bone marrow (or less than 5 blasts out of every 100 blood cells)

> No signs and symptoms of cancer outside the bone marrow (extramedullary disease)

> Cancer has not returned in 4 weeks

In an incomplete blood count recovery (CRi), the platelet count or absolute neutrophil count (ANC) has not yet returned to normal. ANC is an estimate of the body's ability to fight infections, especially bacterial infections.

Phases of treatment

There are 3 phases of treatment: induction, consolidation, and maintenance. However, not all doctors use the same terms when discussing treatment. In general, there are several phases of intense chemotherapy followed by a longer phase of maintenance chemotherapy. The number of phases and the type chemotherapy given depends on the type of leukemia, as well as how your child responds to the first phases of treatment.

Induction
Induction is the first phase of treatment. Your child will likely spend time in the hospital for part of this treatment. Treatment is a multi-drug combination of chemotherapies (called multi-agent chemotherapy) and steroids.

Infants with ALL are usually given one week of steroid treatment to begin induction, and their blood will be checked for a response after the first week of treatment.

The goal of induction is a complete response (CR) or remission. In CR, less than 5% blasts remain at the end of induction. When induction does not lead to a complete response, it is called induction failure. This could be a sign that this cancer is very difficult to treat. How the cancer responds to initial treatment affects prognosis. Treatment following induction failure is often an allogeneic SCT (stem cell transplant). However, a different multi-agent chemotherapy might be tried before an SCT in order to reduce the amount of minimal residual disease.

After induction, your child will have bone marrow tests to look for a complete response and to measure the amount of cancer that might remain (minimal residual disease).

Minimal residual disease

In minimal residual disease (MRD), ALL seems to be in remission after induction, but very sensitive lab tests, such as flow cytometry or PCR, find leukemia cells in your bone marrow. Not all MRD can be found with tests. The aim of treatment will be to reduce the amount of MRD.

What do I need to know?

Parents and caregivers say the induction phase is the most stressful part of treatment. There is uncertainty, fear, and confusion. In addition, there will be a lot of tests, appointments, and disruption to routine. Lastly, you will hear a lot of unfamiliar words to describe a complex disease. Seek out support groups at your local hospital, through social media, or from those listed in the back of this book. Look to friends, relatives, neighbors, and co-workers for social support. Your child or teen will also need a support network. Their network might look different than yours. Support services such as counseling are also available. Ask the treatment team for more information. They are there to help.

Consolidation

Consolidation is the second phase of treatment. It is needed to kill any cancer cells called minimal residual disease (MRD) that might remain after induction.

> It is very important to take medicine on time and exactly as prescribed. Don't miss or skip a dose!

Consolidation lasts 6 to 9 months and aims to prevent cancer from returning. The time spent in consolidation and the intensity of the drug regimen will vary. It will be based on factors such as your age, how well you respond to treatment, and risk factors.

Maintenance

Maintenance chemotherapy is the final, and longest, stage of treatment in childhood ALL. Treatment is less intensive than prior chemotherapy. It usually lasts at least 2 years and is outpatient. The goal is to lower the risk of relapse.

What do I need to know?

It is very important to continue to take your medicine as prescribed and not miss or skip any doses. This helps to prevent relapse. Ask your treatment team for help if you have trouble paying for medicine or trouble remembering to take your medicine.

Prevention and treatment of CNS disease

Treatment to prevent ALL from spreading to the central nervous system (CNS) is called CNS prophylaxis or prophylactic treatment. CNS prophylaxis is typically given throughout the entire course of ALL therapy, from induction, to consolidation, to the maintenance phases of treatment.

All treatment plans include intrathecal (IT) chemotherapy. IT chemotherapy is injected into spinal fluid. Some treatments include intrathecal treatment throughout therapy, whereas others do not include it in maintenance. Options for intrathecal chemotherapy include intrathecal methotrexate or a combination of intrathecal methotrexate, cytarabine, and hydrocortisone (known as triple intrathecal chemotherapy).

CNS relapse

Sometimes ALL travels to or relapses in the CNS. In this case, special treatment is needed. Treatment of CNS disease includes systemic chemotherapy able to penetrate the blood-brain barrier, direct intrathecal chemotherapy, and cranial radiation.

> Treatment is needed to prevent ALL from spreading to the central nervous system (CNS). This is called CNS prophylaxis.

Surveillance and monitoring

Monitoring or surveillance watches for any changes in your child's condition.

For a list and timing of the tests your child might receive, see Guide 4.

Guide 4
Surveillance and monitoring

Surveillance	1 year after treatment →	**Every 1 to 2 months** • Physical exam, including testicular exam • CBC with differential • LFTs until normal
	2 years after treatment →	**Every 3 to 6 months** • Physical exam, including testicular exam • CBC with differential
	3 years or more after treatment ends →	**Every 6 to 12 months** • Physical exam, including testicular exam • CBC with differential
Procedures and molecular testing	Bone marrow aspirate and cerebrospinal fluid (CSF) for suspected relapse • If bone marrow aspirate is done: Flow cytometry with additional studies that may include cytogenetics, FISH, molecular testing, and MRD testing.	
	Consider periodic *BCR-ABL1* testing if Ph+ ALL	
Monitoring for late effects	Echocardiogram as needed	
	Neuropsychological testing as needed	
	Monitor for healthy weight and encourage healthy lifestyle choices given increased risk of obesity in those with history of childhood ALL	
	See *Follow-up Guidelines for Survivors of Childhood, Adolescent, and Young Adult Cancers from the Children's Oncology Group (COG)*: survivorshipguidelines.org	
	See *NCCN Guidelines for Patients: Adolescents and Young Adults with Cancer* found at NCCN.org/patientguidelines	

Relapse

When leukemia returns after a period of remission, it is called a relapse. The goal of treatment is to achieve remission again. Relapse happens in about 1 out of 5 cases. A relapse is very serious. It is important to ask about prognosis.

Those with relapsed ALL are placed into risk groups. Length of first complete remission (CR1) and site of relapse are two important factors. Relapse can occur in the bone marrow called isolated medullary relapse, in areas outside of the marrow or blood such the brain or testicles called isolated extramedullary relapse, or a combination of both. In general, those with a later relapse, 3 or more years after starting treatment, have the best prognosis.

Refractory

When leukemia remains and does not respond to treatment, it is called refractory or resistant cancer. The cancer may be resistant at the start of treatment or it may become resistant during treatment. Refractory disease is very serious. It is important to ask about prognosis.

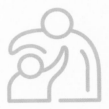

For parents and caregivers

- Take care of yourself. This is a stressful time. Make an appointment to see your doctor. Seek out and ask for support. Support can be a friend, relative, neighbor, or co-worker.

- This will be a confusing time. You will hear a lot of unfamiliar words. Start conversations with questions and about your concerns.

- Encourage your child to interact with their health care team, to ask questions, and to talk about how they feel.

- Teach your teen how and when to take their medicine, what to do if their medicine is low, how to refill a prescription, how to manage side effects, and who to call if they have questions about their medicine or treatment.

- Explain to your child or teen why taking medicine is important. Create a chart so they can keep track of when to take medicine or use an electronic device to schedule a reminder.

- Treating pediatric ALL is complex. Not everyone responds to treatment the same way. Some do better than expected. Others do worse. A treatment response takes time.

- Celebrate treatment milestones and other events. Find ways to engage your child. Explore new interests together.

Review

> The goal of treatment is a complete response.

> Induction is the first stage of treatment. Your child will likely spend time in the hospital for part of this treatment.

> Consolidation or post-induction therapy is the second stage of treatment. It is needed to kill any cancer cells called minimal residual disease (MRD) that might be left after induction. Consolidation usually lasts 6 to 9 months.

> Maintenance or post-consolidation therapy is the final phase of treatment. It usually lasts 2 years.

> Central nervous system (CNS) prophylaxis is given to prevent ALL from spreading to the brain and spinal fluid.

> Monitoring watches for any changes in your child's condition.

> ALL that returns after remission is called relapse. To prevent relapse, it is important to take your medicine as prescribed and not miss or skip any doses.

> When ALL does not respond to treatment or stops responding to treatment, it is called refractory or resistant cancer.

Tips to prepare your child for treatment

✓ Remain relaxed and calm

✓ Explain what to expect

✓ Use simple language

✓ Encourage questions

✓ Answer questions truthfully

✓ It's okay to say, "I don't know"

5
Ph-negative or Ph-like B-ALL

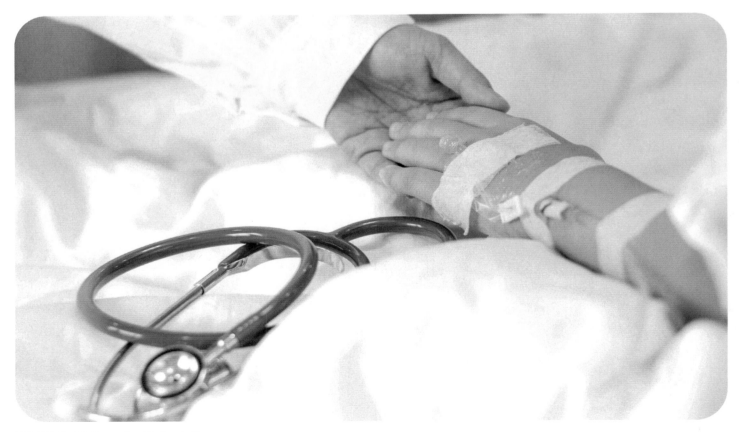

This chapter is for those with Philadelphia chromosome-negative (Ph-) B-ALL or Philadelphia-chromosome-like (Ph-like) B-ALL. A clinical trial is the preferred treatment for both Ph- and Ph-like B-ALL.

Overview

Both Ph-negative (Ph-) and Ph-like B-ALL do not have the Philadelphia chromosome. However, Ph-like B-ALL is very similar to Ph-positive (Ph+) B-ALL. Ph-like cases are by definition *BCR/ABL*-negative, and are also always *MLL-ETV/RUNX1*- and *TCF3/PBX1*-negative. Ph-like ALL is difficult to treat due to the number of possible mutations. It might be referred to as *BCR-ABL1*-like ALL.

Before starting treatment, your child will be placed into a risk group. Risk is based on white blood cell (WBC) count and age at diagnosis.

> Standard risk is for those with a WBC less than 50,000/mm³ and who are between 1 and 10 years of age.

> High risk is for those with a WBC higher than 50,000/mm³ and who are less than 1 year of age or 10 years of age and older.

Induction will either be a clinical trial or chemotherapy. A clinical trial is preferred. All regimens include central nervous system (CNS) prophylaxis with systemic therapy and/or intrathecal (IT) therapy. After induction is complete, your child's risk group will be reassessed before starting consolidation.

Treatment by risk group can be found in Guide 5.

Guide 5
Treatment by risk group: Ph- or Ph-like B-ALL

	Induction		Consolidation
Standard risk • WBC is less than 50,000/mm³ • Between 1 and 10 years of age	Clinical trial (preferred) or chemotherapy	→	Check response before consolidation: • If MRD+, then clinical trial or intensified consolidation chemotherapy. If MRD+ continues, then clinical trial, chemotherapy, blinatumomab, or tisagenlecleucel. • If MRD-, then continue therapy, followed by maintenance and surveillance.
High risk • WBC is 50,000/mm³ or more • Less than 1 year of age or 10 years of age and over	Clinical trial (preferred) or chemotherapy	→	Check response before consolidation: • If MRD+, then clinical trial or intensified consolidation chemotherapy. If MRD+ continues, then clinical trial, chemotherapy, blinatumomab, or tisagenlecleucel. • If MRD-, then continue therapy, followed by maintenance and surveillance.

Ph- treatment

Ph- B-ALL is the most common type of B-ALL.

Induction
Many induction treatment regimens are part of ongoing clinical trials. Induction is a combination of systemic therapies. Systemic therapies work throughout the body. All treatment regimens include systemic and/or intrathecal therapy (injected into the spinal fluid) to prevent CNS disease.

Consolidation
Before starting consolidation, your child will be placed into a risk group. These might include: low risk (LR), standard risk (SR), high risk (HR), or very high risk (VHR). Risk is based on a variety of factors.

Consolidation treatment may be partially based on whether there is minimal residual disease (MRD) at the end of induction. When cancer remains after induction, it is called MRD-positive (MRD+).

Maintenance
Maintenance chemotherapy is given if no minimal residual disease remains (MRD-). A stem cell transplant (SCT) might also be an option. An SCT depends upon donor availability and your child's health at the time of potential SCT.

Ph-like treatment

Ph-like is a category of B-ALL that is classified by genetic changes, and may be considered high risk.

Induction
Many induction treatment regimens are part of ongoing clinical trials. Induction is a combination of therapies. All treatment regimens include systemic and/or intrathecal therapy to prevent CNS disease.

During induction, your child's blood will be tested for genetic mutations. This information is used to choose the best consolidation therapy for your child.

Below are some mutations classified as Ph-like B-ALL that might be targeted during induction:

> *CRLF2*- with *ABL* class kinase fusion

> *CRLF2*+

> *CRLF2*- with *JAK2* fusions

Consolidation
When cancer remains after induction, it is called MRD-positive (MRD+). Depending on the type of Ph-like genetic mutation found, tyrosine kinase inhibitors (TKIs) such as dasatininb or ruxolitinib may be offered to your child in addition to chemotherapy or as part of a clinical trial.

Maintenance
Maintenance chemotherapy is given if no minimal residual disease remains (MRD-). A stem cell transplant (SCT) might also be an option. An SCT depends upon donor availability and your child's health at the time of potential SCT.

MRD+ after induction

Treatment response will be measured after completing induction. The goal is a complete response (CR). In less than a CR, cancer remains. Tests will look for minimal residual disease (MRD). When MRD is found, it is called MRD-positive (MRD+). A certain low level of MRD may be permissible (called a threshold), but it depends on the treatment. Your child's doctor can explain this to you.

Treatment

MRD+ is treated with a clinical trial or intensified consolidation chemotherapy. A clinical trial is preferred. If after consolidation, MRD is negative (MRD-), then your child will continue chemotherapy, followed by maintenance chemotherapy or a stem cell transplant (SCT).

If MRD+ continues after consolidation, options include:

> Clinical trial (preferred)

> Chemotherapy

> Blinatumomab

> Tisagenlecleucel

After the treatment above, SCT can be considered as the next treatment option for those whose MRD becomes negative. If MRD is continuously positive, then treatment might be one from the list above. An SCT depends upon donor availability and your child's health at the time of potential SCT.

Tips for parents and caregivers

✓ Take breaks, exercise, eat, and rest

✓ Ask for help

✓ Let others help

✓ Seek out a support network

✓ Use your support network

✓ Help your child or teen find their own support network

Surveillance and monitoring

During maintenance or after a stem cell transplant, your child will be monitored for signs of recurrence called relapse.

First relapse

First relapse is the return of cancer after a period of remission. The goal of treatment is to achieve remission (a complete response) again. This is not always possible. Treatment options are based on the time from initial diagnosis to relapse and if there is extramedullary disease (cancer outside of the bone marrow and blood).

Cancer can return in the bone marrow called isolated medullary relapse, outside the bone marrow called isolated extramedullary relapse, or a combination of both called combined relapse. Extramedullary relapse is cancer found in the central nervous system or testicles.

Isolated extramedullary relapse requires systemic therapy to prevent relapse in bone marrow. Likewise, isolated medullary relapse requires intrathecal treatment to prevent cancer in the central nervous system.

Treatment for B-ALL first relapse will be based on your prior therapy and length of time from initial diagnosis to relapse. Most treatment paths lead to an SCT. Treatment options for first relapse are found in Guide 6.

Guide 6
Early or late first relapse treatment options: B-ALL

Treatment	Consolidation	
	Check response before consolidation	
	If CR with MRD-, then • Clinical trial (preferred) • Blinatumomab (for early first relapse) • Chemotherapy	→ If early first relapse, then SCT If late first relapse, then • Maintenance chemotherapy or • Consider SCT
• Clinical trial (preferred) or • Systemic therapy →	If CR with MRD+, then • Clinical trial (preferred) • Chemotherapy • Blinatumomab • Tisagenlecleucel • Inotuzumab (not FDA approved in children)	→ SCT
	Less than CR, see multiple relapse or refractory disease	

Early and late first relapse

Early relapse is defined as follows:

> Less than 36 months (3 years) from initial diagnosis for isolated or combined bone marrow relapse OR

> Less than 18 months from initial diagnosis for isolated extramedullary relapse

Late relapse is defined as follows:

> 36 months (3 years) or more from initial diagnosis for isolated or combined bone marrow relapse OR

> 18 months or more from initial diagnosis for isolated extramedullary relapse

First relapse after SCT

Treatment options for a relapse that occurs after a stem cell transplant (SCT) include:

> Clinical trial (preferred)

> Chemotherapy

> Blinatumomab

> Tisagenlecleucel

> Inotuzumab ozogamicin (not FDA approved for children)

Treatment response will be checked before starting consolidation.

> If there is a complete response, then a second SCT might follow.

> If less than a complete response, then treatment might be one from the list above.

The goal is to achieve an MRD-negative result before an SCT. However, in some cases an SCT might be considered in those who are MRD+. An SCT depends upon donor availability and your child's health at the time of potential SCT.

Multiple relapse or refractory

Relapse can happen more than once. With each relapse the goal of treatment is a complete response or remission. When cancer returns only in the bone marrow, it is called isolated medullary relapse. When cancer is found in the central nervous system and testicles, but not in the bone marrow or blood, it is called isolated extramedullary relapse. In this case, systemic therapy is needed to prevent relapse in bone marrow. When leukemia remains and does not respond to treatment, it is called refractory. Treatment for multiple relapse or refractory disease can be found in Guide 7.

Treatment options include:

> Clinical trial (preferred)

> Chemotherapy

> Blinatumomab

> Tisagenlecleucel

> Inotuzumab ozogamicin (not FDA approved for children)

Treatment response will be checked before starting consolidation.

> If there is a complete response, then a stem cell transplant (SCT) will follow.

> If less than a complete response, then treatment might be an alternative therapy and/or best supportive or palliative care.

Guide 7
Multiple relapse or refractory disease: Ph- or Ph-like B-ALL

	Treatment	Consolidation
Multiple relapse or Refractory disease	• Clinical trial (preferred) • Chemotherapy • Blinatumomab • Tisagenlecleucel • Inotuzumab (not FDA approved in children)	→ Check response before consolidation: • If complete response, then SCT • If less than a complete response, then alternative therapy and/or best supportive care and palliative care

Review

> - Both Ph-negative (Ph-) and Ph-like B-ALL do not have the Philadelphia chromosome. However, Ph-like B-ALL is very similar to Ph-positive (Ph+) B-ALL. Ph- B-ALL is the most common type of B-ALL.

> - Induction is a combination of systemic therapies. A clinical trial is the preferred treatment.

> - All treatment regimens include systemic and/or intrathecal (IT) therapy to prevent central nervous system (CNS) disease.

> - When cancer remains after induction, it is called MRD-positive (MRD+).

> - MRD+ is treated with a clinical trial (preferred) or intensified consolidation chemotherapy.

> - During maintenance or after a stem cell transplant, your child will be monitored for signs of recurrence called relapse.

> - First relapse is the return of cancer after a period of remission. The goal of treatment is to achieve remission again. A clinical trial is the preferred treatment.

> - Relapse can happen more than once. With each relapse the goal of treatment is a complete response or remission.

> - Treatment after a complete response is often a stem cell transplant (SCT). However, an SCT depends upon donor availability and your child's health at the time of potential SCT.

An important note about teens

✓ Teens are less likely to take their medicine. Help your teen feel in control by finding a routine that works for them.

✓ Talk to your teen about how to refill prescriptions and what to do so they don't run out of medicine.

6
Ph-positive B-ALL

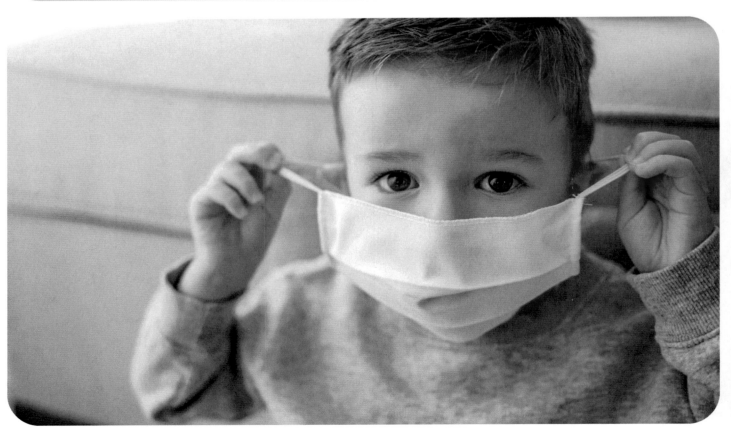

In Ph-positive (Ph+) B-ALL, tests show the presence of the Philadelphia chromosome. This happens when a piece of chromosome 9 and a piece of chromosome 22 break off and trade places with each other. The result is a fused gene called *BCR-ABL1*. Treatment is usually an intensive combination of systemic therapies.

Treatment

Ph+ B-ALL is less common than other types of B-ALL. Treatment aims to stop the activity of the BCR-ABL fusion protein. Although Ph+ B-ALL is considered high risk, there are effective treatments such as imatinib, a tyrosine kinase inhibitor (TKI) that targets the BCR-ABL fusion protein, and other TKIs such as dasatinib, nilotinib, and ponatinib. Treatment is usually an intensive combination of systemic therapies. Systemic therapies work throughout the body.

Induction
There are 2 induction options:

> Clinical trial with a TKI (preferred)

> Chemotherapy with a TKI

All regimens include central nervous system (CNS) prophylaxis with systemic therapy and/or intrathecal (IT) therapy.

> A clinical trial is recommended for anyone with ALL.

After completing induction, your child will be placed into a risk group.

> In standard risk, your child had a complete response, although a small amount of minimal residual disease (MRD) may remain.

> In high risk, your child had less than a complete response and/or a higher amount of MRD remains.

Consolidation

Consolidation treatment options can be found in Guide 8.

> For standard risk, consolidation is a continuation of chemotherapy with a TKI

> For high risk, consolidation options include a clinical trial (preferred), continuation of chemotherapy with a TKI, blinatumomab, or tisagenlecleucel

Maintenance

Maintenance is given to prevent the return or spread of ALL. It is usually a continuation of treatment, but might be at a lower dose. A stem cell transplant (SCT) might be an option. An SCT depends upon donor availability and your child's health at the time of potential SCT.

> For standard risk, maintenance might be a continuation of chemotherapy with a TKI or an SCT.

> For high risk, maintenance might be an SCT followed by a TKI.

Surveillance

During maintenance or after a stem cell transplant, your child will be monitored for signs of recurrence.

Guide 8
Treatment by risk group: Ph+ B-ALL

	Consolidation	Maintenance
Standard risk • Low minimal residual disease (MRD) found	Continue chemotherapy with TKI →	Maintenance therapy with TKI ――― Consider SCT
High risk • Less than complete response (CR) • MRD found at end of induction	Clinical trial (preferred) ――― Continue chemotherapy with TKI ――― Blinatumomab ――― Tisagenlecleucel	→ SCT → Consider TKI after SCT

Relapsed or refractory disease

Relapse is the return of cancer after a period of remission. The goal of treatment is to achieve remission again. Cancer can return in the bone marrow called isolated medullary relapse, outside the bone marrow called isolated extramedullary relapse, or a combination of both (combined relapse). Extramedullary relapse can occur in the central nervous system or testicles.

Mutation testing will be done before starting treatment. Treatment options for Ph+ B-ALL relapse are found in Guide 9.

Treatment options include:

> Clinical trial (preferred)

> Chemotherapy

> Backbone chemotherapy with TKI

> Some regimens for Ph- B-ALL may be considered for Ph+ ALL with TKIs

> Consider dasatinib or imatinib

> Blinatumomab

> Tisagenlecleucel

> Inotuzumab ozogamicin (not FDA approved for children)

Guide 9
Relapse or refractory disease: Ph+ B-ALL

	Treatment	Consolidation
Multiple relapse or Refractory disease	• Clinical trial (preferred) • Chemotherapy • Backbone chemotherapy with TKI • Some regimens for Ph- B-ALL may be considered for Ph+ B-ALL with TKIs • Consider dasatinib or imatinib • Blinatumomab • Tisagenlecleucel • Inotuzumab (not FDA approved in children)	Check response before consolidation: • If complete response, then SCT • If less than a complete response, then alternative therapy and/or best supportive care and palliative care

Most treatment paths lead toward a stem cell transplant (SCT). The goal is to achieve an MRD-negative result before an SCT. If less than a complete response, then treatment options include an alternative therapy and/or best supportive or palliative care. In some cases an SCT might be considered in those who are MRD+. An SCT depends upon donor availability and your child's health at the time of potential SCT.

Multiple relapse

B-ALL can relapse multiple times. With each relapse the goal of treatment is a complete response (CR). This is not always possible.

Refractory

When leukemia remains and does not respond to treatment, it is called refractory or resistant. The cancer may be resistant at the start of treatment or it may become resistant during treatment. Refractory disease is very serious. It is important to ask about prognosis. Treatment options are the same as for relapse.

Review

> In Ph-positive (Ph+) B-ALL, tests show the presence of the Philadelphia chromosome.

> The goal of treatment is a complete response and to prevent the spread of cancer to areas outside the blood.

> Treatment is usually an intensive combination of systemic therapies. All regimens include central nervous system (CNS) prophylaxis with systemic therapy and/or intrathecal (IT) therapy.

> Relapse is the return of cancer after a period of remission. The goal of treatment is to achieve remission (a complete response) again.

> For multiple relapse or refractory disease, the goal is to achieve an MRD-negative result before a stem cell transplant (SCT). An SCT is not an option for everyone.

> An SCT depends upon donor availability and your child's health at the time of potential SCT.

7
T-ALL

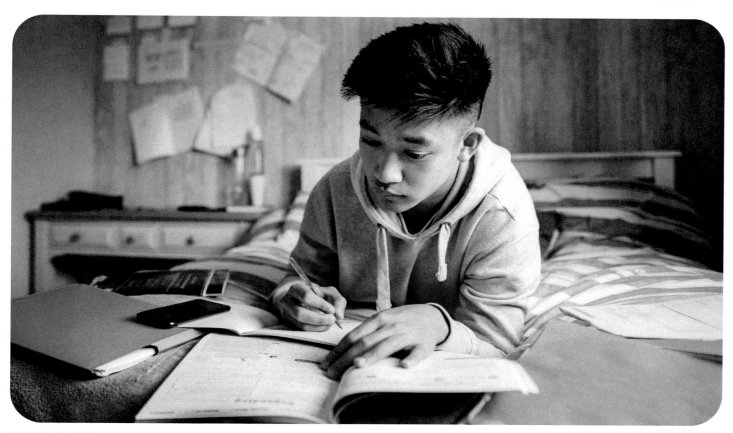

T-ALL includes a group of cancers that start in T-cell lymphocytes. T-ALL is less common than B-ALL. Treatment options include a clinical trial or chemotherapy.

Treatment

It is recommended that T-ALL be treated in a clinical trial when possible.

Induction
There are 2 induction options:

> Clinical trial (preferred)

> Chemotherapy

All regimens include central nervous system (CNS) prophylaxis with systemic therapy and/or intrathecal (IT) therapy. Treatment response will be measured after completing induction. Tests will look for minimal residual disease (MRD).

Consolidation
Consolidation is a continuation of chemotherapy. After consolidation, treatment response will be assessed. If MRD remains, then your child will be placed into a very high-risk group. For risk group definitions, see Guide 10.

Continuation therapy
The goal of extended maintenance or continuation therapy is to prevent cancer from returning (called a relapse) or spreading to the central nervous system (CNS) or testicles, and to reduce the amount of minimal residual disease (MRD). After continuation therapy, a stem cell transplant might be an option. However, an SCT depends upon donor availability and your child's health at the time of potential SCT. For continuation therapy, see Guide 11.

Guide 10
T-ALL risk groups after induction

Very high risk	• MRD after consolidation is more than 0.1%
High risk	• Absence of standard and very high-risk features
Standard risk	• On day 29, MRD is less than 0.01%, no cancer is found in central nervous system or testicles, and there is no steroid pretreatment

Surveillance

After a complete response or a stem cell transplant, your child will be monitored for signs of recurrence or relapse. Relapse is the return of cancer.

Relapse

T-ALL often returns within 2 years of diagnosis.

First relapse

When cancer returns after remission, it is called relapse. Relapse can occur in the bone marrow called isolated medullary relapse, in the testicles or central nervous system called isolated extramedullary relapse, or a combination of both. Isolated extramedullary relapse requires systemic therapy to prevent relapse in bone marrow.

Treatment options for a first relapse:

- ➤ Clinical trial (preferred)
- ➤ Chemotherapy
- ➤ TKI for *ABL*-class translocation

Treatments will likely include a combination of drugs. If relapse is more than 3 years after initial diagnosis, then your doctor might consider treatment using the same induction regimen again.

Complete response

If treatment causes a complete response (CR), then you will continue with this treatment. The next step would be a stem cell transplant (SCT).

Less than complete response

If treatment does not cause a complete response, then a different treatment will be tried. It might be a clinical trial or chemotherapy.

Multiple relapse

Relapse can happen multiple times. With each relapse the goal of treatment is a complete response.

Treatment options include:

- ➤ Clinical trial (preferred)
- ➤ Chemotherapy

Guide 11
T-ALL continuation therapy after consolidation

Very high risk	• Clinical trial (preferred) • Continue chemotherapy • Alternative therapy	➡ Consider SCT
Standard or high risk	Continue chemotherapy	

Treatment response will be checked before starting consolidation.

> If there is a complete response, then a stem cell transplant (SCT) will follow.

> If less than a complete response, then treatment might be an alternative therapy and/or best supportive or palliative care.

The goal is to achieve an MRD-negative result before an SCT. However, in some cases an SCT might be considered in those who are MRD+.

Refractory

When leukemia remains and does not respond to treatment, it is called refractory or resistant. The cancer may be resistant at the start of treatment or it may become resistant during treatment. Refractory disease is very serious. It is important to ask about prognosis. Refractory treatment options can be the same as for multiple relapse.

Review

> T-ALL includes a group of cancers that start in T-cell lymphocytes. T-ALL is less common than B-ALL.

> It is recommended that T-ALL be treated in a clinical trial when possible. Chemotherapy is also a treatment option. All regimens include central nervous system (CNS) prophylaxis with systemic therapy and/or intrathecal (IT) therapy.

> The goal of treatment is a complete response (CR).

> After a CR or a stem cell transplant (SCT), your child will be monitored for signs of recurrence or relapse.

> When cancer returns or relapses, treatment is a clinical trial (preferred) or chemotherapy. The goal of treatment is to have another CR. After a CR, an SCT might follow. An SCT depends upon donor availability and your child's health at the time of potential SCT.

> Cancer may be resistant at the start of treatment or it may become resistant during treatment. This is called refractory.

8
Infant ALL

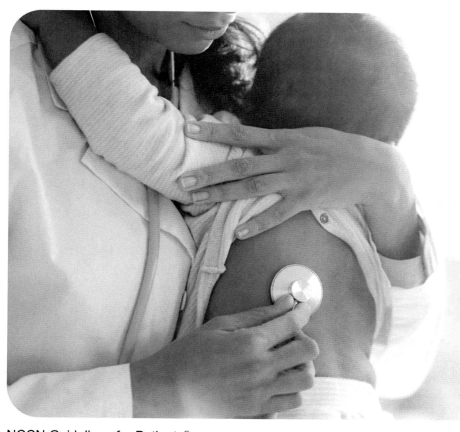

ALL treatment for infants is different than other age groups. Infants are children under 12 months of age.

Interfant induction

Interfant regimens are those used for infants. You do not have to be enrolled in a clinical trial to have Interfant induction. However, enrolling in a clinical trial may be the best choice for your child.

There are 2 treatment options:

> Clinical trial (preferred)

> Interfant induction

Interfant induction is a multi-drug therapy that might include prednisone, dexamethasone, vincristine, cytarabine, daunorubicin, pegaspargase, or methotrexate. Other systemic therapies might be used. All regimens include central nervous system (CNS) prophylaxis with systemic therapy and/or intrathecal (IT) therapy. Systemic therapy works throughout the body. IT therapy is injected into the spinal fluid.

Consolidation

After diagnosis, your child's bone marrow will be tested to look for genetic changes and minimal residual disease. Consolidation is based on *KMT2A* status (11q23). If *KMT2A* is found, it is called *KMT2A*-rearranged. There are 2 risk groups for *KMT2A*-rearranged: high or intermediate. See Guide 12.

KMT2A-rearranged
For *KMT2A*-rearranged, consolidation will be Interfant intensive chemotherapy. After consolidation, disease response may be checked again.

Guide 12 Risk group features: Infant	
High risk	• *KMT2A*-rearranged; and • Less than 3 months of age with any WBC or less than 6 months of age with WBC 300,000 or higher; or • Remains MRD+ after intensive consolidation therapy (any age and WBC)
Intermediate risk	• *KMT2A*-rearranged and not high risk
Standard risk	• Not *KMT2A*-rearranged

The next treatment options include:

> For high risk, a stem cell transplant (SCT) may be considered or maintenance chemotherapy

> For intermediate risk, maintenance chemotherapy is the option

Not *KMT2A*-rearranged

Consolidation treatment options include:

> Clinical trial

> Chemotherapy based on risk groups similar to other Ph- B-ALL children (non-infants)

> Interfant consolidation

Interfant consolidation is multi-drug treatment. A clinical trial or chemotherapy will also likely include multi-drug therapy. The goal of consolidation is to reduce the amount of minimal residual disease (MRD).

> If MRD-, then maintenance therapy will follow.

> If MRD+, treatment will continue in order to reduce MRD. A stem cell transplant (SCT) may be an option.

Maintenance

Maintenance chemotherapy is given to prevent the return or spread of ALL. It is usually a continuation of treatment, but might be at a lower dose.

Surveillance

During maintenance or after a stem cell transplant, your child will be monitored for signs of recurrence called relapse. If cancer returns, treatment can be found under B-ALL or T-ALL first relapse.

Review

> Infants are children under 12 months of age.

> There are special treatment regimens for infants.

> Treatment options include a clinical trial, multi-drug therapy chemotherapy, and possibly a stem cell transplant (SCT).

> All regimens include central nervous system (CNS) prophylaxis with systemic therapy and/or intrathecal (IT) therapy.

> Consolidation is based on *KMT2A* status (11q23).

> Maintenance chemotherapy is given to prevent the return or spread of ALL.

> During maintenance or after a stem cell transplant, your child will be monitored for signs of recurrence called relapse.

9
Making treatment decisions

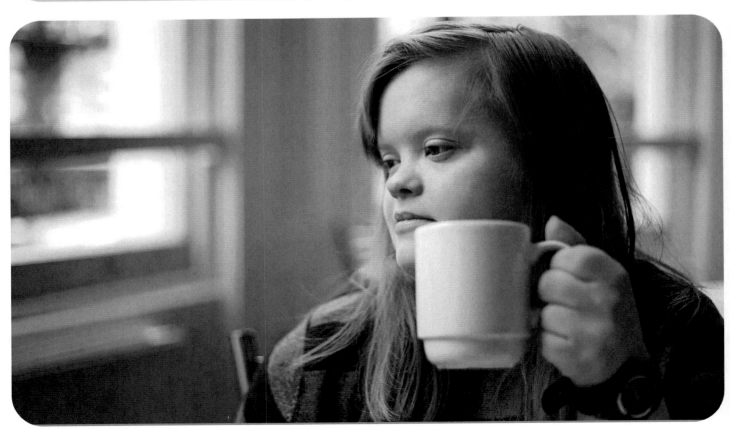

It's important to be comfortable with the cancer treatment you choose. This starts with having an open and honest conversation with your child and their doctor.

It's your choice

In shared decision-making, you and your doctors share information, discuss the options, and agree on a treatment plan. It starts with an open and honest conversation between you and your doctor.

Treatment decisions are very personal. What is important to you may not be important to someone else.

Some things that may play a role in your decision-making:

> What you want and how that might differ from what others want

> Your religious and spiritual beliefs

> Your feelings about certain treatments like surgery or chemotherapy

> Your feelings about pain or side effects such as nausea and vomiting

> Cost of treatment, travel to treatment centers, and time away from school or work

> Quality of life and length of life

> How active you are and the activities that are important to you

Think about what you want from treatment. Discuss openly the risks and benefits of specific treatments and procedures. Weigh options and share concerns with your doctor. If you take the time to build a relationship with your doctor, it will help you feel supported when considering options and making treatment decisions.

Second opinion

It is normal to want to start treatment as soon as possible. While cancer can't be ignored, there is time to have another doctor review your test results and suggest a treatment plan. This is called getting a second opinion, and it's a normal part of cancer care. Even doctors get second opinions!

Things you can do to prepare:

> Check with your insurance company about its rules on second opinions. There may be out-of-pocket costs to see doctors who are not part of your insurance plan.

> Make plans to have copies of all your records sent to the doctor you will see for your second opinion.

Support groups

Many people diagnosed with cancer find support groups to be helpful. Support groups often include people at different stages of treatment. Some people may be newly diagnosed, while others may be finished with treatment. If your hospital or community doesn't have support groups for people with cancer, check out the websites listed in this book.

Questions to ask your doctors

Possible questions to ask your doctors are listed on the following pages. Feel free to use these questions or come up with your own. Be clear about your goals for treatment and find out what to expect from treatment.

Questions to ask about diagnosis and testing

1. What subtype of pediatric ALL does my child have? What does this mean in terms of prognosis and treatment options?

2. What tests are needed? What other tests do you recommend?

3. How soon will we know the results and who will explain them to us?

4. Where will the tests take place? How long will the tests take?

5. Is there a cancer center or hospital nearby that specializes in this type and subtype of cancer?

6. What will you do to make my child comfortable during testing? Should I be in the room?

7. How do we prepare for testing? How will the test be done? How can I talk to my child about what to expect?

8. Would you give us a copy of the pathology report and other test results?

9. Who will talk with us about the next steps? When?

10. Will treatment start before the test results are in?

11. How many bone marrow tests are needed? When are they done?

12. Are there any resources you would recommend that can help me explain to my child what is happening?

Questions to ask about options

1. What will happen if we do nothing?

2. How do age, white blood cell (WBC) count, health, and other factors affect the options?

3. How will treatment affect my child's fertility? Should we see a fertility specialist before starting treatment?

4. Is my child a candidate for a blood stem cell transplant?

5. Is my child a candidate for a clinical trial?

6. Which option is proven to work best for my child's ALL subtype, age, and other risk factors?

7. Does any option offer a cure or long-term cancer control? Are the chances any better for one option than another? Less time-consuming? Less expensive?

8. How do you know if treatment is working? How will we know if treatment is working?

9. What are our options if the treatment stops working?

10. Are there any life-threatening side effects of this treatment? How will these be monitored?

11. What should we expect from this treatment? How long will treatment last?

12. Can we stop treatment at any time? What will happen? How will we know when to stop blood transfusions or antibiotics?

Questions to ask about treatment

1. What are the treatment choices? What are the benefits and risks?

2. Which treatment do you recommend and why?

3. How long do we have to decide?

4. Will we have to go to the hospital or elsewhere for treatment? How often? How long is each visit? Will we have to stay overnight in the hospital or make travel plans?

5. Do we have a choice of when to begin treatment? Can we choose the days and times of treatment?

6. How much will the treatment hurt? What will you do to make my child comfortable?

7. How much will this treatment cost? What does my insurance cover? Are there any programs to help pay for treatment?

8. What kind of treatment will we do at home? What can we do to prepare our home to ensure our child's safety or the safety of other family members in the household?

9. What can we do to prevent or relieve side effects? What will you do?

10. Which treatment will give my child the best quality of life? Which treatment will extend life? By how long?

11. Will my child miss school? Be able to play with friends?

12. What in particular should be avoided or taken with caution while receiving treatment?

_____

_____

_____

_____

_____

Questions to ask your doctors about their experience

1. What is your experience treating this subtype of pediatric ALL?

2. What is the experience of those on your team?

3. Do you only treat pediatric ALL? What else do you treat?

4. I would like to get a second opinion. Is there someone you recommend?

5. I would like another pathologist or hematopathologist to review the blood samples. Is there someone you recommend?

6. How many patients like my child (of the same age, gender, race) have you treated?

7. Will you be consulting with pediatric ALL experts to discuss my child's care? Who will you consult?

8. How many procedures like the one you're suggesting have you done?

9. Is this treatment a major part of your practice?

10. How many of your patients have had complications? What were the complications?

Questions to ask about clinical trials

1. What clinical trials are available? Are we eligible for any of them? Why or why not?

2. What are the treatments used in the clinical trial?

3. What does the treatment do?

4. Has the treatment been used before? Has it been used for other types of cancer?

5. What are the risks and benefits of this treatment?

6. What side effects should we expect? How will the side effects be controlled?

7. How long will my child be on the clinical trial?

8. Will we be able to get other treatment if this doesn't work?

9. How will you know the treatment is working?

10. Will the clinical trial cost me anything? If so, how much?

Questions to ask about stem cell transplants

1. How do you find a donor?

2. How long will we have to wait for a stem cell transplant (SCT)?

3. What do we need to do to prepare?

4. What will you do to prepare?

5. What are the risks to myself and/or the donor?

6. How will the transplant affect my child's prognosis?

7. How will a transplant affect the quality and length of my child's life?

8. What should we expect?

9. How long should my child expect to be in the hospital?

10. How will my child feel before, during, and after the transplant?

11. How many SCTs has this center done for those with this type of pediatric ALL?

12. Will my child have more than one SCT?

13. What side effects may occur after an SCT?

14. Is radiation treatment included with an SCT for my child?

Questions to ask about side effects

1. What are the side effects of treatment?

2. How long will these side effects last? Do any side effects lessen or worsen in severity over time?

3. What side effects should I watch for? What side effects are expected and which are life-threatening?

4. When should I call the doctor? Can I text?

5. What medicines can my child take to prevent or relieve side effects?

6. What can we do to help with pain and other side effects?

7. Will you stop treatment or change treatment if there are side effects? What do you look for?

8. What can we do to lessen or prevent side effects? What will you do?

9. What side effects are life-long and irreversible even after completing treatment?

10. What medicines may worsen side effects of treatment?

Questions to ask about survivorship and late effects

1. What happens after treatment?

2. What are the chances ALL will return or that my child will get another type of cancer?

3. Whom do we see for follow-up care? How often?

4. Should my child see a dentist? An eye doctor?

5. What tests will my child have to monitor their health?

6. What late effects are caused by this treatment? How will these be screened? What should we look for?

7. What should we do if my child has trouble with work or school? Or difficulty focusing?

8. We are looking for a survivor support group. What support groups or other resources can you recommend?

Websites

Alex's Lemonade Stand Foundation
alexslemonade.org

American Association for Clinical Chemistry
labtestsonline.org

American Cancer Society
cancer.org/cancer/leukemia-in-children

American Society of Hematology
hematology.org/education/patients

Be The Match®
bethematch.org

Blood & Marrow Transplant Information Network
bmtinfonet.org

CancerCare
cancercare.org

CancerFree Kids
cancerfreekids.org

Chemocare
chemocare.com

Children's National®
childrensnational.org

Children's Oncology Group
survivorshipguidelines.org

KidsHealth®
kidshealth.org

MedlinePlus
medlineplus.gov

National Bone Marrow Transplant Link
nbmtlink.org

National Cancer Institute
cancer.gov/types/leukemia

cancer.gov/publications/patient-education/children-with-cancer.pdf

National Coalition for Cancer Survivorship
canceradvocacy.org/toolbox/

National Hospice and Palliative Care Organization
nhpco.org/patients-and-caregivers

OncoLink
oncolink.org

Pediatric Cancer Foundation of the Lehigh Valley
pcflv.org

Radiological Society of North America
radiologyinfo.org

Stupid Cancer
stupidcancer.org

The Leukemia & Lymphoma Society

lls.org/leukemia/acute-lymphoblastic-leukemia/childhood-all

U.S. Department of Health & Human Services

bloodstemcell.hrsa.gov

Words to know

absolute neutrophil count (ANC)
An estimate of the body's ability to fight infections, especially bacterial infections.

adolescent and young adult (AYA)
People who are 15 to 39 years of age at the time of initial cancer diagnosis.

acute lymphoblastic leukemia (ALL)
A fast-growing cancer that causes too many immature white blood cells called lymphoblasts to be made.

antibody
A protein made by a plasma cell (a type of white blood cell).

autologous
Stem cells come from you.

allogeneic
Donor that may or may not be related to you.

B cell
A type of lymphocyte.

BCR-ABL1 protein
An abnormal protein that is made by the *BCR-ABL1* fusion gene and causes too many abnormal white blood cells to be made.

biopsy
A procedure that removes tissue samples.

blast
An immature blood cell. Also called lymphoblast.

blood stem cell
An immature blood-forming cell from which all other types of blood cells are made. Also called hematopoietic stem cell.

blood stem cell transplant (SCT)
A treatment that replaces damaged or diseased cells in the bone marrow with healthy blood-forming cells.

bone marrow
The soft, sponge-like tissue in the center of most bones where blood cells are made.

bone marrow aspirate
The removal of a small amount of liquid bone marrow to test for disease.

bone marrow biopsy
The removal of a small amount of solid bone and bone marrow to test for disease.

chemotherapy
Drugs that kill fast-growing cells, including cancer cells and normal cells.

chromosomes
Long strands that contain bundles of coded instructions in cells for making and controlling cells.

clinical trial
A study of how safe and helpful tests and treatments are for people.

computed tomography (CT)
A test that uses x-rays from many angles to make a picture of the insides of the body.

consolidation
The second stage of treatment.

contrast
A substance put into your body to make clearer pictures during imaging tests.

deoxyribonucleic acid (DNA)
Long strands of genetic information found inside cells.

donor
A person who gives their organs, tissues, or cells to another person.

extramedullary
Outside the bone marrow.

gene
Coded instructions in cells for making new cells and controlling how cells behave.

hematopoietic stem cell transplant (HSCT)
A treatment that replaces damaged or diseased cells in the bone marrow with healthy blood-forming cells. Also called stem cell transplant (SCT).

hematopathologist
A doctor who specializes in blood diseases by looking at cells under a microscope.

hematologist
A doctor who's an expert in diseases of the blood.

hereditary
Passed down from parent to child through coded information in cells (genes).

hyperdiploidy
Leukemia cells with 51 to 67 chromosomes.

hypodiploidy
Leukemia cells with fewer than 44 chromosomes.

human leukocyte antigen (HLA)
Special proteins on the surface of cells that help the body to tell its own cells apart from foreign cells.

immune system
The body's natural defense against infection and disease.

immunotherapy
A treatment with drugs that help the body find and destroy cancer cells.

induction
The first stage of treatment.

infant
A child under 12 months of age.

infection
An illness caused by germs.

infusion
A method for delivering chemotherapy into the vein in a controlled manner.

Interfant induction
A cancer treatment for infants (those under 12 months of age).

intravenous (IV)
A method of giving drugs by a needle or tube inserted into a vein.

interventional radiologist
A doctor who is an expert in imaging tests and using image-guided tools to perform minimally invasive techniques to diagnose or treat disease.

leukapheresis
A procedure that separates leukocytes from the blood.

leukemia
A disease in which there are too many white blood cells.

liver function test (LFT)
A lab test that measures chemicals made or processed by the liver.

lymph node
A small, bean-shaped, disease-fighting structure.

lymphoblast
An immature lymphocyte. Also called blast.

lymphocyte
A type of white blood cell that is part of the immune system.

lymphoid
Referring to a type of white blood cell called a lymphocyte.

magnetic resonance imaging (MRI)
A test that uses radio waves and powerful magnets to make pictures of the insides of the body.

medical oncologist
A doctor who is an expert in cancer drugs.

medullary
In the bone marrow.

minimal residual disease (MRD)
Cancer that remains after treatment.

mutation
An abnormal change.

myeloid
Referring to a type of white blood cell called a granulocyte.

myelosuppression
A condition in which bone marrow activity is decreased, resulting in fewer red blood cells, white blood cells, and platelets.

natural killer (NK) cell
A type of lymphocyte.

oncologist
A doctor who is an expert in the treatment of cancer.

palliative care
Health care that includes symptom relief but not cancer treatment. Also sometimes called supportive care.

pathologist
A doctor who is an expert in testing cells and tissue to find disease.

pediatric
People who are 18 years of age or under at the time of initial diagnosis.

peripheral blood
Blood that circulates throughout the body.

pharmacogenomic
The study of how genes affect a person's response to drugs.

Philadelphia chromosome (Ph)
An abnormal, short chromosome 22 that is formed when parts of chromosomes 9 and 22 switch with each other. The result is the *BCR-ABL1* fused gene.

physical exam
A study of the body by a health expert for signs of disease.

platelet
A type of blood cell that helps control bleeding. Also called thrombocyte.

polymerase chain reaction (PCR)
A lab process in which copies of a piece of DNA are made.

positron emission tomography (PET)
A test that uses radioactive material to see the shape and function of body parts.

predisposition syndrome
Certain genetic changes, or mutations, can increase a person's chances of developing cancer.

prognosis
The likely course and outcome of a disease.

progression
The growth or spread of cancer after being tested or treated.

radiation therapy (RT)
A treatment that uses high-energy rays.

radiologist
A doctor who is an expert in imaging tests.

recurrence
The return of cancer after a cancer-free period.

red blood cell (RBC)
A type of blood cell that carries oxygen from the lungs to the rest of the body. Also called an erythrocyte.

refractory
A cancer that does not improve with treatment.

relapse
The return or worsening of cancer after a period of improvement.

regimen
A treatment plan that includes specific information about drug dose, when medicine is taken, and how long treatment will last.

remission
There are minor or no signs of a disease.

resistance
When cancer does not respond to a drug treatment.

scrotal ultrasound
Uses sound waves to make images of the scrotum. The scrotum is the pouch of skin at the base of the penis that contains the testicles.

side effect
An unhealthy or unpleasant physical or emotional response to treatment.

stem cell transplant (SCT)
A cancer treatment that destroys bone marrow and the replaces it by adding healthy blood stem cells. Also called hematopoietic stem cell transplant (HSCT) or bone marrow transplant (BMT).

steroid
A drug used to reduce redness, swelling, and pain, but also to kill cancer cells.

subtype
A smaller group within a type of cancer that is based on certain cell features.

supportive care
Health care that includes symptom relief but not cancer treatment. Also called palliative care or best supportive care.

surveillance
Testing that is done after treatment ends to check for the return of cancer.

systemic therapy
Treatment that works throughout the body.

T cell
A type of lymphocyte.

targeted therapy
A drug treatment that targets and attacks specific cancer cells.

translocation
When pieces of two chromosomes (long strands of coded instructions for controlling cells) break off and switch with each other.

tumor lysis syndrome (TLS)
A condition caused when waste released by dead cells is not quickly cleared out of the body.

tumor marker
A substance found in body tissue or fluid that may be a sign of cancer.

white blood cell (WBC)
A type of blood cell that helps fight infections in the body. Also called a leukocyte.

NCCN Contributors

This patient guide is based on the NCCN Clinical Practice Guidelines in Oncology (NCCN Guidelines®) for Pediatric Acute Lymphoblastic Leukemia. It was adapted, reviewed, and published with help from the following people:

Dorothy A. Shead, MS
Director, Patient Information Operations

Laura J. Hanisch, PsyD
Medical Writer/Patient Information Specialist

Erin Vidic, MA
Medical Writer

Rachael Clarke
Senior Medical Copyeditor

Tanya Fischer, MEd, MSLIS
Medical Writer

Kim Williams
Creative Services Manager

Susan Kidney
Design Specialist

The NCCN Guidelines® for Pediatric Acute Lymphoblastic Leukemia Version 1.2021 were developed by the following NCCN Panel Members:

Patrick Brown, MD/Chair
The Sidney Kimmel Comprehensive Cancer Center at Johns Hopkins

*Hiroto Inaba, MD, PhD/Vice-Chair
St. Jude Children's Research Hospital/ The University of Tennessee Health Science Center

*Colleen Annesley, MD
Fred Hutchinson Cancer Research Center/ Seattle Cancer Care Alliance

Jill Beck, MD
Fred & Pamela Buffett Cancer Center

*Susan Colace, MD
The Ohio State University Comprehensive Cancer Center - James Cancer Hospital and Solove Research Institute

Mari Dallas, MD
Case Comprehensive Cancer Center/ University Hospitals Seidman Cancer Center and Cleveland Clinic Taussig Cancer Institute

Satiro De Oliveira, MD
UCLA Jonsson Comprehensive Cancer Center

Kenneth DeSantes, MD
University of Wisconsin Carbone Cancer Center

Kara Kelly, MD
Roswell Park Comprehensive Cancer Center

Carrie Kitko, MD
Vanderbilt-Ingram Cancer Center

Norman Lacayo, MD
Stanford Cancer Institute

Luke Maese, DO
Huntsman Cancer Institute at the University of Utah

Kris Mahadeo, MD, MPH
The University of Texas MD Anderson Cancer Center

Ronica Nanda, MD
Moffitt Cancer Center

Valentina Nardi, MD
Massachusetts General Hospital Cancer Center

Vilmarie Rodriguez, MD
Mayo Clinic Cancer Center

Jenna Rossoff, MD
Robert H. Lurie Comprehensive Cancer Center of Northwestern University Ann & Robert H. Lurie Children's Hospital of Chicago

*Laura Schuettpelz, MD, PhD
Siteman Cancer Center at Barnes- Jewish Hospital and Washington University School of Medicine

Lewis Silverman, MD
Dana-Farber Cancer Institute

Jessica Sun, MD
Duke Cancer Institute

David Teachey, MD
Abramson Cancer Center at the University of Pennsylvania - Children's Hospital of Philadelphia

Julie Wolfson, MD, MSHS
O'Neal Comprehensive Cancer Center at UAB

*Victor Wong, MD
UC San Diego Moores Cancer Center - Rady Children's Hospital of San Diego

Gregory Yanik, MD
University of Michigan Rogel Cancer Center

NCCN Staff

Jennifer Burns, MS
Manager, Guidelines Support

Ndiya Ogba, PhD
Oncology Scientist/Senior Medical Writer

* Reviewed this patient guide.
For disclosures, visit NCCN.org/about/disclosure.aspx.

NCCN Cancer Centers

Abramson Cancer Center
at the University of Pennsylvania
Philadelphia, Pennsylvania
800.789.7366 • pennmedicine.org/cancer

Fred & Pamela Buffett Cancer Center
Omaha, Nebraska
402.559.5600 • unmc.edu/cancercenter

Case Comprehensive Cancer Center/
University Hospitals Seidman Cancer
Center and Cleveland Clinic Taussig
Cancer Institute
Cleveland, Ohio
800.641.2422 • UH Seidman Cancer Center
uhhospitals.org/services/cancer-services
866.223.8100 • CC Taussig Cancer Institute
my.clevelandclinic.org/departments/cancer
216.844.8797 • Case CCC
case.edu/cancer

City of Hope National Medical Center
Los Angeles, California
800.826.4673 • cityofhope.org

Dana-Farber/Brigham and
Women's Cancer Center
Boston, Massachusetts
617.732.5500
youhaveus.org

Massachusetts General Hospital
Cancer Center
617.726.5130
massgeneral.org/cancer-center

Duke Cancer Institute
Durham, North Carolina
888.275.3853 • dukecancerinstitute.org

Fox Chase Cancer Center
Philadelphia, Pennsylvania
888.369.2427 • foxchase.org

Huntsman Cancer Institute
at the University of Utah
Salt Lake City, Utah
800.824.2073
huntsmancancer.org

Fred Hutchinson Cancer
Research Center/Seattle
Cancer Care Alliance
Seattle, Washington
206.606.7222 • seattlecca.org
206.667.5000 • fredhutch.org

The Sidney Kimmel Comprehensive
Cancer Center at Johns Hopkins
Baltimore, Maryland
410.955.8964
hopkinskimmelcancercenter.org

Robert H. Lurie Comprehensive
Cancer Center of Northwestern
University
Chicago, Illinois
866.587.4322 • cancer.northwestern.edu

Mayo Clinic Cancer Center
Phoenix/Scottsdale, Arizona
Jacksonville, Florida
Rochester, Minnesota
480.301.8000 • Arizona
904.953.0853 • Florida
507.538.3270 • Minnesota
mayoclinic.org/cancercenter

Memorial Sloan Kettering
Cancer Center
New York, New York
800.525.2225 • mskcc.org

Moffitt Cancer Center
Tampa, Florida
888.663.3488 • moffitt.org

The Ohio State University
Comprehensive Cancer Center -
James Cancer Hospital and
Solove Research Institute
Columbus, Ohio
800.293.5066 • cancer.osu.edu

O'Neal Comprehensive
Cancer Center at UAB
Birmingham, Alabama
800.822.0933 • uab.edu/onealcancercenter

Roswell Park Comprehensive
Cancer Center
Buffalo, New York
877.275.7724 • roswellpark.org

Siteman Cancer Center at Barnes-
Jewish Hospital and Washington
University School of Medicine
St. Louis, Missouri
800.600.3606 • siteman.wustl.edu

St. Jude Children's Research Hospital
The University of Tennessee
Health Science Center
Memphis, Tennessee
866.278.5833 • stjude.org
901.448.5500 • uthsc.edu

Stanford Cancer Institute
Stanford, California
877.668.7535 • cancer.stanford.edu

UC San Diego Moores Cancer Center
La Jolla, California
858.822.6100• cancer.ucsd.edu

UCLA Jonsson
Comprehensive Cancer Center
Los Angeles, California
310.825.5268 • cancer.ucla.edu

UCSF Helen Diller Family
Comprehensive Cancer Center
San Francisco, California
800.689.8273 • cancer.ucsf.edu

University of Colorado Cancer Center
Aurora, Colorado
720.848.0300 • coloradocancercenter.org

University of Michigan
Rogel Cancer Center
Ann Arbor, Michigan
800.865.1125 • rogelcancercenter.org

The University of Texas
MD Anderson Cancer Center
Houston, Texas
844.269.5922 • mdanderson.org

University of Wisconsin
Carbone Cancer Center
Madison, Wisconsin
608.265.1700 • uwhealth.org/cancer

UT Southwestern Simmons
Comprehensive Cancer Center
Dallas, Texas
214.648.3111 • utsouthwestern.edu/simmons

Vanderbilt-Ingram Cancer Center
Nashville, Tennessee
877.936.8422 • vicc.org

Yale Cancer Center/
Smilow Cancer Hospital
New Haven, Connecticut
855.4.SMILOW • yalecancercenter.org

Notes

Made in the USA
Middletown, DE
16 September 2021